VAGUS NERVE

*Easy Self-Help Exercises to
Overcome Anxiety, Depression,
Trauma, Chronic Diseases and
Finally Improve Your Life*

© Copyright 2019 by LAYNE KELLY
All rights reserved

This document is geared towards providing exact and reliable information with regard to the topic and issue covered. The publication is sold with the idea that the publisher is not required to render accounting, officially permitted or otherwise qualified services. If advice is necessary, legal, or professional, a practiced individual in the profession should be ordered. From a Declaration of Principles which was accepted and approved equally by a Committee of the American Bar Association and a Committee of Publishers and Associations.

In no way is it legal to reproduce, duplicate, or transmit any part of this document in either electronic means or in printed format. Recording of this publication is strictly prohibited and any storage of this document is not allowed unless with written permission from the publisher. All rights reserved.

The information provided herein is stated to be truthful and consistent, in that any liability, in terms of inattention or otherwise, by any usage or abuse of any policies, processes, or directions contained within is the solitary and utter responsibility of the recipient reader. Under no circumstances will any legal responsibility or blame be held against the publisher for any reparation, damages, or monetary loss due to the information herein, either directly or indirectly.

Respective authors own all copyrights not held by the publisher.

The information herein is offered for informational purposes solely and is universal as so. The presentation of the information is without a contract or any type of guarantee assurance.

The trademarks that are used are without any consent, and the publication of the trademark is without permission or backing by the trademark owner. All trademarks and brands within this book are for clarifying purposes only and are owned by the owners themselves, not affiliated with this document

TABLE OF CONTENTS

INTRODUCTION 1

CHAPTER 1: The Vagus Nerve 21

What happens when the vagus nerve isn't working admirably? 25

Unlock the Powers of the Vagus Nerve 31

CHAPTER 2: Function of Vagus Nerve and Polyvagal Theory 39

Vagus Nerve Function 41

Vagus Nerve Stimulation: How to Stimulate the Vagus Nerve Naturally 48

Polyvagal Hypothesis 60

Polyvagal Theory 68

CHAPTER 3: Diseases and Disorders Associated with Vagus Nerve 75

What Causes Vagus Nerve Disorders? 80

Medications for Vagus Nerve Disorders 86

CHAPTER 4: Vagus Nerve and Social Engagement 95

The Social Engagement System 96

Craniosacral Therapy 101

CHAPTER 5: Tapping into the Power of the Vagus Nerve 109

The Autonomic Nervous System (ANS) 110

The Vagal Brake and Social Behavior 119

CHAPTER 6: Exercise and Stimulation 125

Vagus Nerve Stimulation Exercises 126

Meditation - Mindfulness 131

Yoga and Tai Chi 135

CHAPTER 7: Diet and Vagus Nerve 139

Nourishments for Making Acetylcholine 140

Healthy Daily Routines for Vagus Nerve 143

CONCLUSION 155

INTRODUCTION

Vagus nerves also called X or tenth cranial nerve is the most prolonged and generally complex of the cranial nerves. The Vagus nerve originates from the brain through the face and thorax, to the ventral part of the abdomen. It's a blended nerve containing parasympathetic filaments. The vagus nerve has two tactile ganglia (masses of nerve tissue that transmit tangible driving forces): the predominant and the mediocre ganglia. The parts of the predominant ganglion innervate the skin in the concha of the ear. The substandard ganglion emits two branches: the pharyngeal nerve and the prevalent laryngeal nerve. The repetitive laryngeal nerve branches from the vagus in the lower neck and upper thorax to innervate the muscles of the larynx (voice box). The vagus additionally radiates cardiovascular, esophageal, and aspiratory branches. In the stomach area, the vagus innervates most of the stomach-related tract and other stomach viscera.

The vagus nerve has the broadest dissemination of the cranial nerves. Its pharyngeal and laryngeal branches transmit engine driving forces to the pharynx and larynx; its cardiovascular branches act to slow the pace of heartbeat; its bronchial branch acts to contract the bronchi; and its esophageal branches control automatic muscles in the throat, stomach, gallbladder, pancreas, and small digestive system, animating peristalsis and gastrointestinal emissions.

The Vagus nerve incitement, in which the nerve is invigorated with heartbeats of power, is sometimes utilized for patients with epilepsy or melancholy that is generally untreatable; the procedure has additionally been investigated for conditions such as Alzheimer malady and headache.

Cranial Nerves are a significant piece of the human body, as these nerves partake in a considerable most of the things we can do individually, for example, seeing, eating, and such like. These nerves emerge from the cerebrum or brainstem and exist two by two.

They supply blood and sustenance to different organs in the head and the neck zones aside from the vagus nerve, which has an alternate capacity. There are 12 cranial nerves, and larger parts of them convey tangible strands. However, some cranial nerves convey engine filaments also and some convey both tactile and engine filaments.

Among the 12 cranial nerves, there are only 2 nerves that emerge from the cerebellum, while the rest emerge from the brainstem. These cranial nerves have been named dependent on their capacities and structure. Outlined underneath are the rundown of the cranial nerves and their capacities in detail.

As expressed above, there are 12 cranial nerves. These cranial nerves are:

Olfactory Nerve

As the name proposes, this nerve manages the feeling of smell; the receptors of these nerves are situated in the nasal mucosa. This is the most limited nerve among the entirety of the cranial nerves and it doesn't enter the brainstem.

Optic Nerve

Again, as the name recommends, this nerve manages vision; meaning, what we can see and not see. This nerve emerges from the retina of the eye and sends visual signs to the cerebrum, which frames an image of the objects we see. This nerve is viewed as a piece of the fringe sensory system. Any harm or damage to this nerve can prompt a total loss of vision either briefly or forever relying upon the damage caused to the nerve.

Oculomotor Nerve

The Oculomotor Nerve comes third in the rundown of the 12 cranial nerves pursued by the olfactory and the optic nerve. The capacity of this cranial nerve is to control eyeball and eyelid development. This nerve has two-engine part, which have their own particular capacities and are physical engine segment and instinctive engine segment.

Trochlear Nerve

This is otherwise called Cranial Nerve IV and it's the fourth in the rundown of cranial nerves. This is the main cranial nerve that emerges dorsally from the cerebrum. This nerve additionally gives its support to the eye. The principle capacity of this nerve is to give it the capacity to roll the eyes here and there and furthermore outwards.

Trigeminal Nerve

The trigeminal nerve is one of most significant cranial nerves. It has three branches to be specific; these are the ophthalmic, maxillary, and mandibular. Each branch interfaces nerves from the mind to the various pieces of the face. The primary capacity of the trigeminal nerve is to give sensations to the mouth, teeth, face, and the nasal hole. This nerve likewise controls the nerve that enables us to bite in nourishment.

Abducens Nerve

This nerve is likewise called as Cranial Nerve VI. The principle capacity of this cranial nerve is to permit development of the eyes sideways significance away from the nose. Any damage to this nerve can bring about an individual having obscured or twofold vision.

Facial Nerve

The facial nerve is likewise called as Cranial Nerve VII. It has to be two elements in specific, of which one is to convey tactile sign from the tongue to the inside part of the mouth and furthermore this nerve helps an individual produce outward appearance.

Vestibulocochlear Nerve

As the name proposes, this cranial nerve has functions of incorporating two pieces, of which initially is the feeling of hearing, which is the cochlear part and the second is simply the capacity of a person to adjust himself or herself, which shapes the vestibular part. Any harm or damage to this cranial nerve may bring about loss of hearing or offset issues with the influenced person.

Glossopharyngeal Nerve

The Glossopharyngeal Nerve is the ninth cranial nerve that is available in the body. This nerve begins from the brainstem, navigates through the base of the skull, and ends at the mouth in the mucous organs and base of the tongue.

This nerve has different branches; these are the tonsillar branch, tympanic branch, stylopharyngeal branch, carotid sinus nerve branch, and the lingual branch. Since it partitions into numerous branches, then it must have different capacities.

It gets tactile filaments from the pieces of the tongue, carotids, tonsils, and the center ear. It likewise innervates the parasympathetic filaments that help in assimilation and resting of the body. It additionally innervates the engine strands of the stylopharyngeus muscle, which helps in gulping.

Vagus Nerve

This cranial nerve is the longest of every cranial nerve and starts from the brainstem, crosses right down to the mid-region passing the heart, lungs, and throat in transit.

This cranial nerve shapes a piece of the automatic sensory system and controls the body strategies, which are not in the control of an individual like controlling the pulse and supporting in nourishment assimilation. Incitement of the vagus nerve is a favored treatment for patients with epilepsy and melancholy.

Incitement of the vagus nerve because of eruption of the body to specific upgrades prompts a condition called vasovagal syncope or blacking out scenes, as this incitement causes a drop in circulatory strain and pulse.

Adornment Nerve

This is the eleventh cranial nerve of the 12 that exist in the human body. This nerve controls the development of the muscles of the neck. There are two pieces of the Accessory Nerve, which are the spinal and cranial divisions, of which the cranial subdivision is ignored. The spinal adornment nerve gives capacity to the sternocleidomastoid muscle, the upper back, and the shoulder. Any brokenness of this cranial nerve may prompt the shoulders and neck not performing to the ideal level.

Hypoglossal Nerve

The Hypoglossal Nerve is the remainder of the cranial nerves. The fundamental capacity of this cranial nerve is to control developments of the tongue. This nerve begins in the brainstem, navigates through the carotid supply route and jugular vein, and winds up underneath the tongue. Any harm or damage to the hypoglossal nerve may make the tongue totally incapacitated bringing about instance where the individual would not be able to eat or talk appropriately. There are numerous and various causes, which can harm the hypoglossal nerve, for example, a contamination or damage to the nerve bringing about the tongue being incapacitated.

Autonomic sensory system and enteric sensory system

The autonomic sensory system manages an assortment of body process that happens without cognizant exertion. The autonomic framework is the relevant part of the fringe sensory system that is answerable for controlling automatic body capacities, for example, heartbeat, blood stream, breathing, and assimilation.

The Structure of the Autonomic Nervous System

This framework is additionally separated into three branches, namely: the thoughtful framework, the parasympathetic framework, and the enteric sensory system.

- The thoughtful division of the autonomic sensory system directs the flight-or-battle reactions. This division likewise performs such assignments as loosening up the bladder, accelerating pulse, and expanding student's eye.
- The parasympathetic division of the autonomic sensory system helps keep up with the ordinary body capacities and rations physical assets. This division additionally performs such errands as controlling the bladder, hindering pulse, and tightening eye understudies.
- The autonomic sensory system is additionally comprised of a third part, known as the enteric sensory system, which is bound to the gastrointestinal tract.

The autonomic sensory system works by accepting data from the earth and from different pieces of the body. The thoughtful and parasympathetic frameworks will in general have contradicting activities in which one framework will animate a reaction and where the other will hinder it.

Generally, incitement has been thought to happen through the thoughtful framework while restraint was thought to happen by means of the parasympathetic framework. Anyway, numerous special cases to this have been found.

For instance, the thoughtful sensory system will act to raise pulse, while the parasympathetic sensory system will act to bring down it. The two frameworks work in relation to deal with the body's reactions relying on the circumstance and need. In the event that, for instance, you are confronting a danger and need to escape, the thoughtful framework will rapidly assemble your body to make a move. When the danger has passed, the parasympathetic framework will at that point begin to hose these reactions, gradually restoring your body to its typical, resting state.

What Does the Autonomic Nervous System Do?

The autonomic framework controls an assortment of inward procedures including:

- Digestion
- Blood pressure
- Heart rate
- Urination and crap
- Pupillary reaction
- Breathing (respiratory) rate
- Sexual reaction
- Body temperature
- Metabolism
- Electrolyte balance
- Production of body liquids including sweat and salivation
- Emotional reactions

The autonomic nerve pathways associate with various organs to the cerebrum stem or spinal line. There are additionally two key synapses, or compound flagbearers, that are significant for correspondence inside the autonomic sensory system:

- Acetylcholine is regularly utilized in the parasympathetic framework to have a repressing impact.
- Norepinephrine regularly works inside the thoughtful framework to affect stimulatingly the body.

How the Autonomic Nervous System Works

At the point when the parasympathetic and thoughtful parts of the autonomic sensory systems become out of match, individuals can encounter an autonomic issue, likewise called dysautonomia.

There are various kinds of autonomic issue, each with its very own interesting arrangement of side effects, including:

- Acute autonomic loss of motion
- Afferent baroreflex disappointment

- Idiopathic orthostatic hypotension
- Multiple framework decay
- Orthostatic hypotension
- Postprandial hypotension
- Pure autonomic disappointment
- Familial dysautonomia (Riley-Day disorder)
- Secondary orthostatic hypotension

These scatters can happen alone, or because of different conditions, that causes disturbance in the autonomic sensory system, including:

- Autoimmune malady
- Alcohol or medication misuse
- Diabetes
- Parkinson's malady
- Cancer
- Chronic exhaustion disorder
- Peripheral neuropathy
- Aging
- Spinal line issue
- Trauma

Symptoms

If you or somebody you love is encountering disturbances in the autonomic sensory system, you may encounter at least one of the accompanying manifestations. A few people experience one bunch of manifestations one after another and another arrangement of side effects on different occasions. The manifestations can be short-lived and eccentric or activated by explicit circumstances or activities, as in the wake of ingesting certain nourishments or subsequent to standing up rapidly.

- Dizziness or tipsiness after standing
- Fatigue and idleness
- Erectile brokenness
- Lack of sweat or lavish perspiring
- Urinary incontinence
- Difficulty purging the bladder
- Lack of pupillary reaction
- Disturbing a throbbing painfulness
- Faintness (or even genuine blacking out spells)

- Tachycardia (quick pulse)
- Hypotension Gastrointestinal manifestations
- Numbness and shivering
- Severe tension or misery

Enteric sensory system

The enteric sensory system is really a second cerebrum that numerous individuals never realized they had. Even though it has not been experimentally demonstrated and contemplated up until recently as of late, we have all had the experience of having certain premonitions about a circumstance or of having butterflies in our stomach when we are anxious about something. Nevertheless, notwithstanding the fact that these sentiments alongside different stomach related manifestations, we've not paid attention to it as well; we are currently finding out that, the cells and tissues in our stomach really have "a brain of their own" and that we should start paying attention to its messages more.

One of the intriguing things that were found when concentrating on the enteric framework was that, similar synapses that are available in the cerebrum moved to the gut also. By discovering that synthetic concoctions, for example, serotonin, dopamine, glutamate, and norepinephrine are situated inside our enteric sensory system, doctors and researchers have had no real option except to recognize the way that there is some genuine premise to our premonitions and responses that have, up until this point, been genuinely difficult to clarify. These discoveries have approved these "hunches," yet they additionally assume a significant job in helping us explore our very own lives just as in treating different issues of the stomach related tract.

Although our enteric framework makes up a subsequent cerebrum, this doesn't imply that the two structures are working as isolated substances. Actually, the two cerebrums are connected intensely and influence each other in numerous respects. This implies that feeling anxious or being placed in an unpleasant or awkward circumstance will unavoidably cause some piece of intestinal pain and that issues in our stomach can cause a lot of mental uneasiness too. In view of the potential ramifications of the enteric sensory system and what we ordinarily consider as our cerebrum, these two zones of the body should be contemplated independently just as related to each other.

Despite the fact that there is still a lot to find out about our enteric sensory system, we can at present utilize the ebb and flow, looking into in reducing intestinal and mental trouble, just as helping us to run our lives even more beneficially. By realizing that our hunches are similarly as substantial as any thoughts that we think of intelligently, we can really tune in to the data given to us by our enteric framework. On the other side, we can use our brain to help mend issues happening in our stomach related tract.

CHAPTER 1:

The Vagus Nerve

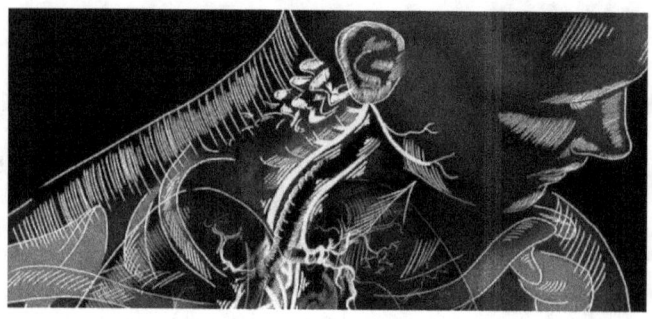

As said, the vagus nerve is one of the two cranial nerves that are incredibly long, reaching out from the mind stem, right to the viscera. The vagus nerves convey a wide arrangement of sign to and from the mind, and they are liable for various natural reactions in the body. You may likewise hear the vagus nerve called Cranial Nerve X, as it is the tenth cranial nerve or the Wandering Nerve. A lot of research has been done on the vagus nerve, as it is an entrancing cranial nerve.

Vagus is Latin for "meandering," and it is an exact portrayal of this nerve, which rises at the back of the skull and wanders in a comfortable manner through the mid-region, with various stretching nerves encountering the heart, lungs, voicebox, stomach, and ears, among other body parts. The vagus nerve conveys approaching data from the sensory system to the mind, giving data about what the body is doing, and it likewise transmits active data, which administers a scope of reflex reactions.

The vagus nerve directs the heartbeat, control muscle development, keeps the individual breathing, and transmit an assortment of synthetics through the body. It is likewise liable for keeping the stomach-related tract in working request, getting the muscles of the stomach and digestion tracts to help process nourishment, and sending back data about what is being processed and what the body is receiving in return.

At the point when the vagus nerve is invigorated, the reaction is frequently a decrease in pulse or relaxing. Now and again, unreasonable incitement can make somebody have what is known as a vaso-vagal reaction, seeming to fall into a blackout or extreme lethargies since their pulse and circulatory strain drop to such an extent. Particular incitement of this nerve is likewise utilized in some medicinal treatment; vagus incitement seems to profit individuals who experience the ill effects of sorrow, for instance, it is additionally once in a while used to treat epilepsy.

You typically don't see the activities of the privilege and left vagus nerves, yet you presumably would see if this nerve stopped working because of infection or injury, in light of the fact that the vagus nerve is one of the numerous crucial nerves which keeps your body in working request. Without the elements of the vagus nerve, you would see that it's hard to talk, inhale, or eat, and your pulse would turn out to be incredibly unpredictable.

We can separate the elements of the vagus nerve into four key zones:

Parasympathetic

This is liable for substantial capacities while we are very still. Consider things like assimilation, metabolic procedures, and pulse. It has likewise been portrayed as the "bolster and breed" or "rest and overview" framework for its job in salivation, sexual excitement, processing, and pee.

Sensory

This process tangible data from the heart, lungs, stomach area, and throat

Motor

The vagus nerve gives development to the neck muscles that are liable for discourse and gulping.

Special tangible

It gives taste sensation behind the tongue.

There are numerous imperative capacities that are affected by the vagus nerve, for instance; keeping a consistent pulse, breathing, perspiring, managing circulatory strain and blood glucose, advancing kidney capacity, and ripeness. It sends data about the condition of your internal organs to your cerebrum. Essentially, it is assisting with significant capacities that keep us alive.

What happens when the vagus nerve isn't working admirably?

A little examination into the vagus nerve finds an entire host of conditions that have either been emphatically connected or are as of now being explored for a connect to the nerve. These range from minor inconveniences to significant issues. Obviously, on the off chance that you are affected anywhere on a range, it can influence your general sentiment of prosperity and general execution.

The vast majority will encounter a vasovagal reaction because of a stressor or overstimulation of the vagus nerve sooner or later. Circulatory strain brings down pulse, eases back, and the veins in your legs broaden, which can cause sickness or blacking out. This is a, for the most part, an innocuous reaction which leaves without anyone else, be that as it may, a few people who experience it all the more incessantly may need to look for restorative assistance.

Some different issues connected with vagus nerve brokenness include stoutness, tension, temperament issue, bradycardia, gastrointestinal infections, incessant irritation, swooning, and seizures.

Obviously, the greater part of these conditions illustrated can prompt further ailment, for instance, corpulence and aggravation are both connected with diseases and diabetes. Tension or mindset issue may likewise prompt despondency.

How does "hacking" the vagus work?

There is a developing assortment of research to recommend that we can control or "hack" the vagus nerve. Vagus hacks go back to some research directed in the year 1998. Through this work, it was found that by invigorating the vagus nerve with an electrical drive could decrease the body's incendiary reaction.

This has positive ramifications for the treatment conditions, for example, Crohn's Disease, rheumatoid joint inflammation, and other incendiary infections. Tracey's exploration frames the premise of the thought for bioelectronics, which we currently observe when treating the condition. for example, discouragement and epilepsy.

Outside of those conditions, aggravation is a reaction that we as a whole have in our bodies, regularly because of stress. For certain individuals, pressure and fiery reaction can get incessant, prompting other medical problems.

The vagus nerve is connected to such a significant number of various capacities, that there are more "hacks" than having a bioelectric gadget embedded to animate it (this is typically just for extraordinary cases). Truth be told, specialists have discovered that we can battle aggravation by connecting with the vagus nerve and improving "vagal tone," like an exercise!

How about we take a gander at what you can be doing:

Work on your passionate wellbeing

A recent report found that a high vagal tone was a piece of a criticism circle between physical wellbeing, positive feelings, and positive social associations. These elements influence each other with a self-supporting dynamic.

During the examination, members utilized Loving Kindness Meditation (LKM) as an approach to affect emphatically their passionate wellbeing. The analysts likewise found out that when individuals thought about positive social associations or attempted to improve their bonds with different people, it beneficially affected vagal tone.

Work on gut wellbeing

Did you realize that "hunch" is a genuine article? A sign from the vagus nerve go from the gut to the cerebrum. This has been connected to regulating state of mind and a few sorts of dread and uneasiness. An indication of a solid vagal tone is somebody who has elegance, under strain characteristic that most business visionaries could utilize!

Your vagus nerve is continually sending refreshed tangible data about the condition of your body's organs, stomach-related tract, pulse, and other data, up to your mind by means of various nerves. There is research to show that our gut organisms and those pathways to the cerebrum are interlinked. It is likewise imagined that gut microbiota are the potential key modulator of the invulnerable and the sensory systems. In this manner, keeping up a solid gut is a vagus "hack."

The takeaway: Gut wellbeing differs from individual to individual and relies upon how you are manufactured, yet by and large, you can take probiotics, eat sound, have adjusted eating routine of entire nourishments, evade pointless utilization of anti-infection agents, and moderate utilization of sugary food sources or liquor. As a further note, while probiotics are yet being investigated for their potential, a Canadian report saw them as a viable PTSD treatment. There are additional suggestions for the treatment of stress - investigating whether you can profit by taking them might be a straightforward advance you can take.

The vagus nerve assumes a fundamental job in our general wellbeing and prosperity. As a businessperson, you've presumably felt the impacts of the physiological reactions it oversees without acknowledging it – especially during distressing periods.

"Hacking" your vagus nerve is extremely about embracing a couple of solid practices that keep it invigorated and working ideally. There are more procedures we could plunge into, yet those recorded are the absolute least, difficult to execute and have strong logical sponsorship. You can take full breaths from your office!

In the event that you do happen to experience the ill effects of one of the more constant incendiary conditions, vagus nerve incitement through electrical driving forces shows a great deal of guarantee. This might be something to examine and rise with your medicinal expert.

Unlock the Powers of the Vagus Nerve

The vagus nerve shouldn't be stunned into shape. It can likewise be conditioned and fortified like a muscle. Here are some outstanding practices you can do that may improve your wellbeing notably:

Positive Social Relationships

An examination had members contemplate, others while quietly, rehashed positive expressions about loved ones, contrasted with the controls. The meditators demonstrated a general increment in positive feelings like peacefulness, satisfaction, and expectation subsequent to finishing the class. These positive musings of others prompted an improvement in the vagal capacity as found in pulse inconstancy. The outcomes likewise demonstrated a more conditioned vagus nerve than when pondering.

Cold

Cold presentation, for example, cool showers, or face dunking animates the nerve also.

Studies show that when your body changes with chilly, your battle or flight (thoughtful) framework decays, your rest, condensation (parasympathetic) framework increments, and this are intervened by the vagus nerve. Any sort of intense cold presentation including drinking super cold water will build vagus nerve initiation.

Swishing

Another home solution for an under-invigorated vagus nerve is to rinse the body with water. Washing really invigorates the muscles of the bed, which are terminated by the vagus nerve.

"Ordinarily, patients will destroy a piece, which is a decent sign and on the off chance that they don't, we prescribe that they do it normally, then consistently until they see that they do fire destroying a piece," says Hoffman. "This has been appeared to promptly improve working memory execution."

Singing and Chanting

Humming, mantra reciting, song singing, and peppy vivacious singing, all expand pulse fluctuation (HRV) in somewhat various ways. Basically, singing resembles starting a vagal siphon conveying loosening up waves. Singing as loud as possible works the muscles in the back of the throat to actuate the vagus. Singing as one, this is regularly done in houses of worship and synagogues, additionally builds HRV and vagus work. Singing has been found to build oxytocin, otherwise called the adoration hormone, since it makes individuals feel more like each other.

Backrub

You can invigorate your vagus nerve by rubbing your feet and your neck along the carotid sinus, situated along the carotid veins on either side of your neck. A neck and back rub can help diminish seizures. A foot rub can bring down your pulse and circulatory strain. A weight back rub can likewise enact the vagus nerve. These back rubs are utilized to assist newborn children with putting on weight by invigorating gut work, to a great extent, intervened by initiating the vagus nerve.

Chuckling

Happiness and giggling are common resistant promoters. Giggling likewise invigorates the vagus nerve. Research shows how chuckling expands HRV in a gathering domain.

There are different case reports of individuals blacking out from giggling, and this might be from the vagus nerve/parasympathetic framework being animated excessively. Blacking out can come after giggling just as pee, hacking, gulping, or solid discharge - which are all aided along by vagus enactment.

Yoga & Tai Chi

Both have increment on vagus nerve action and your parasympathetic framework when all is said and done. Studies have demonstrated that yoga builds GABA, a quieting synapse in your mind. Scientists trust it does this by "invigorating vagal afferents (filaments)," which increment movement in the parasympathetic sensory system. This is particularly useful for individuals who battle with uneasiness or misery. Studies show that jujitsu additionally can 'upgrade vagal adjustment.'

Breathing Deeply & Slowly

Your heart and neck contain neurons that have receptors called baroreceptors, which identify the circulatory strain and transmit the neuronal sign to your cerebrum. This enacts your vagus nerve that associates with your heart to bring down circulatory strain and pulse. Slow breathing, with a generic equivalent measure of time taking in and out, expands the affectability of baroreceptors and vagal enactment. Breathing around 5-6 breaths for every moment in the normal grown-up can be exceptionally useful.

Exercise

Exercise expands your cerebrum's development hormone, bolsters your mind's mitochondria, and helps switch psychological decay. On the other hand, it's been appeared to animate the vagus nerve, which prompts valuable cerebrum and psychological well-being impacts. Gentle exercise additionally invigorates the gut stream, which is interceded by the vagus nerve.

Espresso Enemas

Enemas resembles run for your vagus nerve. Growing the gut builds vagus nerve enactment, as it finished with douches. This purging is cultivated by expanding the liver's ability to detoxify poisons in the blood and restricting them to the bile. All the while, the liver purges itself as it discharges the dangerous bile into the little, at that point huge, digestive tract for clearing. The whole blood supply courses through the liver at regular intervals. By holding the espresso 12 to 15 minutes, the blood will circle four to multiple times for purifying, much like a dialysis treatment. The water substance of the espresso invigorates the intestinal peristalsis and discharges the internal organ with the aggregated poisonous bile.

Electrical Wave Stimulation

There are wearable items that send a delicate electrical wave through the left ear channel to animate the body's vagus nerve while synchronizing with music, which thusly invigorates the arrival of synapses in the cerebrum that create a quieting sensation all through the body.

Unwind

Learning how to chill might be the No. 1 thing to help keep your vagus nerve conditioned. As indicated by Hoffman, most loosening up exercises will animate the vagus nerve.

CHAPTER 2:

Function of Vagus Nerve and Polyvagal Theory

People have an Autonomic Nervous System (ANS) that is really included three separate subsystems, the Parasympathetic Nervous System (PNS), the Sympathetic Nervous System (SNS) and the Enteric Nervous System (ENS). The enteric sensory system has been depicted as a "second mind," which speaks with the focal sensory system (CNS) through the parasympathetic (e.g., by means of the vagus nerve) and thoughtful sensory systems. In any case, vertebrate examinations show that when the vagus nerve is cut off, the enteric sensory system keeps on working.

We presently realize that the ENS isn't only equipped for self-sufficiency yet additionally influences the cerebrum. Indeed, around 90 percent of the signs going along the vagus nerve come not from above, yet from the ENS, and that is the reason many consider it as a rcinforcement mind focused on our sun-powered plexus. Our gut senses are not dreams but genuine apprehensive signs that guides quite a bit of our lives.

Our vagus nerve gives the entryway between the two pieces of the autonomic frameworks. The vagus goes about as a bio-educational information transport that courses our motivations going in two ways. Since the vagus nerve goes about as the focal switchboard, it should not shock anyone that debilitated working of this one nerve can prompt such huge numbers of various conditions and issues. Some neurological infections really come up from the gut, spreading to the cerebrum by means of the vagus nerve.

The vagus nerve is the president with regards to having beauty under strain. The autonomic sensory system contains two perfect inverse frameworks that make a reciprocal back-and-forth. This enables your body to look after homeostasis (inward soundness). The thoughtful sensory system is outfitted to fire you up like the gas pedal in a car – it blossoms with adrenaline and cortisol and it's a piece of the battle or flight reaction. The parasympathetic sensory system is the total inverse. The vagus nerve is directional fundamentally for the capacity of the parasympathetic sensory system. Lamentably, the vagus nerve's reflexive reactions can reverse discharge and divert it from companion into saboteur.

Vagus Nerve Function

The vagus nerve has a broad capacity in the body and it is situated all through the chest area. The long cranial nerve is that vagus nerve that associates the mind to the gut.

The vagus nerve additionally helps the heart and your interior organs to work appropriately. Poorly vagal nerve connects frequently with stomach related issues, poor rest wellbeing, exhaustion, and nervousness.

We would glance in more in details at how the vagus nerve capacities and how vagal tone can influence your wellbeing.

Vagus nerve work in the mind

Your vagal nerve assumes a significant job in how your brain functions.

Specialists have discovered that the vagus nerve is the principal association between the cerebrum and gastrointestinal tract and sends data about the condition of the internal organs to the mind. Studies show that vagus nerve work is likewise associated with mental conditions.

Specialists from the Mayo Clinic states that overseeing epilepsy is one reason why there are gadgets to animate the vagal nerve. The animating impact on the vagus nerve sends a sign to the cerebrum and can diminish the recurrence of seizures.

Vagus nerve work and your mind-set

Since your vagal tone is firmly associated with your mind work, it isn't astounding that your vagus nerve influences your mind-set.

Neuroscientists agreed in 2018 upon the poor capacity of the vagus nerve, that it could prompt the mind-set and tension issues. At times, it is conceivable to animate the vagus nerve by improving your gut wellbeing. The expansion in vagal tone can likewise help direct pressure and lighten restless emotions.

Vagus nerve influences your gut wellbeing

Stress and nervousness frequently cause stomach-related miracle because of the manner in which the vagus nerve interfaces the cerebrum and gut.

Specialists call the capacity of the vagus nerve the "gut-cerebrum hub." Stress represses the vagus nerve capacity and influences your stomach-related wellbeing. This vagal brokenness can prompt different stomach related issues brought about by aggravation and poor gut microbiota.

Sometimes, animating the vagus nerve in the gut utilizing probiotics could be a novel method to improve vagal tone. This can treat manifestations of vagus nerve brokenness, for example, bad-tempered inside disorder (IBS) and fiery gut illness (IBD).

Then again, invigorating the vagus nerve work in the mind through unwinding procedures, profound breathing, or intercession can positively affect your gut's wellbeing.

Different examinations have demonstrated that vagus incitement ensures there is sufficient stomach corrosive for processing. Vagus nerve work additionally influences levels of an inborn factor (a kind of protein known as though) in your gut, which is expected to counteract a nutrient B12 lack.

Vagus nerve capacity and craving

The impact of vagus nerve work on your stomach-related framework can likewise control your hunger.

The diary Gastroenterology reports that vagus movement assumes a job in managing your craving. Analysts have discovered that one of the vagus nerve harm manifestations is weight.

Different examinations point to the way that an appropriately working vagus nerve additionally builds sentiments of satiety. Your vagal tone transports sign to your cerebrum, making you feel fuller and may help keep you from gorging.

Be that as it may, scientists clarify that the vagus nerve work is incredibly mind-boggling and confused, and there is little proof to propose that vagus nerve incitement treats corpulence or lower body weight.

Vagus nerve work and your interior organs

Your left and right vagus nerves are associated with the greater part of your inward organs and assist them with working appropriately.

For instance, some researchers gave an account of an investigation demonstrating that an expansion in vagus movement can help decrease cardiovascular breakdown. Specialists found that utilizing a gadget to animate the vagus nerve expanded nitric oxygen levels and brought down aggravation. Both of these are significant in boosting heart wellbeing.

Research likewise shows that vagal nerve action influences bladder work.

Solid vagal nerve work is likewise important for the kidneys to work appropriately and channel poisons likewise. Examinations have demonstrated that invigorating the vagus nerve improves blood course through the kidneys.

Vagus nerve work influences aggravation

A significant motivation to ensure that you have great vagal tone is to lessen irritation in your body.

Albeit, momentary irritation is important to treat diseases and help the body recuperate itself. Long haul aggravation can be hindering to your wellbeing. Incessant aggravation has been connected to illnesses, for example, coronary illness, sensitivities, diabetes, and malignant growth.

Concentrates into the manner in which the vagus nerve capacities have demonstrated, that is, it helps lower provocative reactions. Researchers conjectured that improving the vagus nerve capacity could help oversee aggravation related ailments. Preliminaries have demonstrated that expanded vagus nerve action could help oversee confusions related to corpulence, diabetes, immune system conditions, and poor cardiovascular wellbeing.

Vagus Nerve Stimulation: How to Stimulate the Vagus Nerve Naturally

What is vagus nerve incitement and by what means can improve vagal tone help direct many-body capacities?

Researchers state that incitement of the vagal nerve can allude to any procedure to increment vagal action. There are different strategies for invigorating the vagus nerve to help support your wellbeing. For instance, breathing activities, vigorous working out, back rub, and yoga have all appeared to help and improve vagal tone.

A portion of the advantages of invigorating your vagus nerve incorporate bringing down circulatory strain, improving cardiovascular wellbeing, getting a charge out of better rest, diminishing tension, and boosting mental wellbeing.

We should glance in more detail at the logical proof on the different ways you can animate the vagus nerve.

Sprinkling cold water all over or putting a virus sodden washcloth on the back of your neck can cause vagus nerve incitement.

Studies have indicated that being presented to cold temperatures builds vagus action. An intense introduction to the virus discharges certain synapses in the gastrointestinal framework that influence mental wellbeing.

Different examinations have indicated that an expansion in vagus nerve movement brought about by acclimatization to the virus, which helps parasympathetic action. This is the place pulse backs off and muscles in the gastrointestinal tract unwind, once in a while alluded to as the "rest-and-summary" impact.

Murmur or Sing to Stimulate the Vagus Nerve

Singing in the shower, singing in an ensemble, or simply murmuring along to your main tune can advance great wellbeing through vagus nerve incitement.

In a study including adults, vocalists found out that singing in a gathering influences pulse fluctuation. Scientists found that singing requires guided breathing which can influence vagal tone. This sort of breathing improves the vagal reaction and improves prosperity.

Cognizant Breathing Benefits Vagus Nerve Function

Profound breathing activities where you deliberately control air admission and yield can help unwind and animate the vagal reaction.

The diary Frontiers in Psychology detailed that cognizant breathing cause's vagus nerve incitement.

Breathing in profoundly, and afterward breathing out gradually hinders the pulse and lower circulatory strain.

One investigation found out that doing breathing-activities for 15 minutes per day for about fourteen days significantly affected the measure of air individuals with incessant cardiovascular breakdown could breathe out.

Different investigations show that breathing activities decidedly influence the vagal tone and can improve enthusiastic and mental wellbeing.

Yoga Stimulation for the Vagus Nerve

Numerous yoga practices include cognizant, conscious breathing and can improve vagal tone.

An examination including sound grown-ups found out that moderate breathing and getting the throat muscles help to improve vagal reactions. The yoga procedures bring down circulatory strain and reduce tension.

Another way that yoga practices help to animate the vagus nerve is by utilizing "OM" reciting, the vibration that the reciting or murmuring makes, build vagus action and unwinds.

To discover more, just keep reading, as I will explain several other numerous medical issues you can fix by utilizing some straightforward yoga presents, just as this yoga for complete amateurs.

Mellow Exercising for Vagus Nerve Stimulation

Customary physical activity is useful for your cardiovascular wellbeing and helps in supporting vagal activity.

One of the advantages that practicing has on vagus nerve incitement is to your stomach-related wellbeing. Analysts have found that mellow practicing advances sound vagal tone. This invigorates the gastric muscles and prompting better assimilation. Specialists have discovered that invigorating the "gut-mind hub" enables the stomach to process nourishment better.

You can find out about other regular approaches to improve your stomach related wellbeing in the event that you have a blockage or other assimilation issues.

Probiotics Can Affect the Vagus Nerve and Improve Gut Function

You can resolve a large number of indications of vagal brokenness by taking probiotics to improve your gut microbiota.

There are numerous examinations demonstrating that probiotics can support your stomach-related wellbeing. Some portion of the motivation behind why probiotics are useful for your processing is that they invigorate your vagus nerve.

One examination found out that taking Lactobacillus rhamnosus probiotic could improve your gastrointestinal wellbeing. Since your gut's wellbeing likewise influences your state of mind and cerebrum works through the vagus nerve, probiotics can likewise oversee pressure, tension, and sadness.

I will explain some answers concerning the numerous motivations to take probiotics consistently, which sort of probiotics reestablishes gut verdure in the wake of taking anti-infection agents.

Omega-3 Affects Heart Function and the Vagus Nerve

Taking fish oil enhancements can increment vagal movement and positively affect your cardiovascular wellbeing.

There are many studies indicating how omega-3 cases can keep your heart sound, lessen irritation, and emphatically influence your state of mind.

Will taking omega-3 enhancements animate your vagus nerve? One investigation including men, found that taking omega-3 unsaturated fats animated the vagal nerve. Over a 4-month time span, the men had a lower pulse and better recuperation after exercise when normally taking omega-3 enhancements.

Different investigations have indicated that taking omega-3 normally likewise builds pulse changeability and lessens the danger of cardiovascular sickness.

Back rub to stimulate the Vagus Nerve

One of the advantages of having a back rub to assist you with unwinding is that its increments vagal action in your body.

Gadgets intended to animate the vagus nerve are at times used to control epilepsy seizures. Notwithstanding, rubbing the carotid sinus on the sides of your neck can have a comparable impact.

Clinical studies revealed that kneading the carotid sinus could smother seizures as it animates the vagus nerve. Different specialists state that a carotid sinus rubs increments vagal tone.

Physicians reported that a certified therapeutic expert typically completes a carotid sinus rub. Invigorating the vagus nerve in such a manner can decrease a fast heartbeat and lower circulatory strain rapidly.

There are best basic oils to use in a loosening up back rub to help cut your feelings of anxiety down?

Foot Reflexology to Regulate Vagus Nerve Function

Rubbing your feet benefits your general prosperity since it is another approach to animate your vagus nerve.

One little examination found out that foot reflexology increments vagal tone and has numerous advantages for your cardiovascular framework. Rubbing explicit zones of the foot brings down circulatory strain normally and gives advantages to individuals with coronary illness.

Discontinuous Fasting to Improve Vagus Nerve Function

This is one approach to invigorate your vagus nerve normally and advantage your pulse changeability is to fasten it irregularly.

Discontinuous fasting is now and then called the 5:2 eating regimen. This includes eating regularly for 5 days and afterward on 2 non eating days back to back days, having a fractional quick. Calorie consumption for the fasting days ought to be 500 calories for women and 600 calories for men.

Studies have demonstrated that irregular fasting is a compelling method to get more fit and keep up with weight reduction. The impacts of fasting on the vagus nerve influence the yearning hormone ghrelin.

Different investigations have indicated that fasting is an approach to animate the capacity of the vagus nerve.

On the off chance that you need to get in shape rapidly, find out about the advantages of discontinuous fasting to help shed pounds of muscle versus fat.

Different Methods to Stimulate the Vagus Nerve and Affect its Function

There are different approaches to improve vagal tone for better wellbeing and prosperity:

Chuckling animates the vagus nerve

There is some logical support to the platitude that giggling is the best prescription. The diary Alternative Therapies in Health and Medicine distributed an examination on the impacts of yoga snickering on pulse fluctuation. Controlled giggling sessions diminished uneasiness and lift the mind-set.

Serotonin supplements influence vagus nerve work

Taking enhancements, for example, 5-HTP can support serotonin levels in the cerebrum and increment vagal action. Studies have indicated that 5-

HTP supplements help to invigorate the vagus nerve. This can likewise help with bringing down sadness, lessening hypertension, and boosting your state of mind.

Discover what other common fixings help to support levels of serotonin.

Needle therapy to manage the vagus nerve

One reason why needle therapy is useful for your general wellbeing and prosperity is that it invigorates the vagal nerve. Studies have demonstrated that needle therapy manages vagal action and improves your gastrointestinal wellbeing, respiratory framework, and heart wellbeing. The impact of needle therapy in improving vagal tone can likewise ensure against neurodegenerative ailments.

Muscle unwinding to oversee nervousness and increment vagal tone

One approach to improve vagus nerve work is to perform dynamic muscle unwinding.

On examination including individuals under pressure, we found out that muscle unwinding brought down sentiments of stress and uneasiness. Unwinding treatment increments vagal action and gives various medical advantages. The expansion in vagal tone likewise brought down circulatory strain, decline cholesterol, and lower resting pulse.

To perform dynamic muscle unwinding to animate your vagus nerve, start by straining the muscles in your feet and holding for 10 seconds, at that point discharging them. Rehash this for each muscle bunch as you stir your way up to your body. Do this for 20 minutes every day to profit by expanded vagus nerve incitement.

Polyvagal Hypothesis

Imagining cerebrum science can be something like envisioning a sea tempest. In spite of the fact that we can envision a terrible climate, it is hard to envision change in that climate. In any case, Stephen Porges' polyvagal hypothesis gives advisors a valuable image of the sensory system that can control us in our endeavors to support customers.

Porges' polyvagal hypothesis created out of his analyses with the vagus nerve. The vagus nerve serves the parasympathetic sensory system, which is the quieting part of our sensory system mechanics. The parasympathetic piece of the autonomic sensory system adjusts the thoughtful dynamic part, yet it is considerably more nuanced ways than we comprehended before polyvagal hypothesis.

Our three-section sensory system

Before the polyvagal hypothesis, our sensory system was envisioned as a two-section opposing framework, with more actuation flagging not so much quieting but rather more quieting flagging less enactment. Polyvagal hypothesis recognizes a third sensory system reaction usually called the social commitment framework. This is a perky blend of actuation and quieting that works out of extraordinary nerve impact.

The social commitment framework causes us to explore connections. Helping our customers move into the utilization of their social commitment framework enables them to turn out to be increasingly adaptable in their adapting styles.

The two different pieces of our sensory system capacity to assist us with overseeing dangerous circumstances, most instructors are as of now acquainted with the two guard components activated by these two pieces of the sensory system: thoughtful battle or flight and parasympathetic shutdown, now and then called stop or black out. Utilization of our social commitment framework, then again, requires a feeling of wellbeing.

Polyvagal hypothesis encourages us to comprehend that the two parts of the vagus nerve quiet the body, yet they do as such in various manners. Shutdown, or stop or-black out, happens through the dorsal part of the vagus nerve. This response can feel like the exhausted muscles and tipsiness of terrible influenza. At the point when the dorsal vagal nerve closes down the body, it can move us into fixed status or separation. Notwithstanding, influencing the heart and lungs, the dorsal branch influences the body working beneath the stomach and is engaged with stomach related problems.

The central part of the vagal nerve influences the body, working over the stomach. This branch serves the social commitment framework. The ventral vagal nerve hoses the body's routinely dynamic state. Picture controlling a pony as you ride it back to the stable. You would keep on pulling back on and discharge the reins in nuanced approaches to guarantee that the steed keeps up a proper speed. Moreover, the ventral vagal nerve permits enactment in a nuanced way, therefore, offering an unexpected quality in comparison to thoughtful actuation.

Ventral vagal discharge into movement takes milliseconds, though thoughtful initiation takes seconds and includes different compound responses that are much the same as losing the pony's reins. In addition, when the battle or flight substance responses have started, it can take our bodies 10–20 minutes to come back to our pre-battle/pre-flight state. Ventral vagal discharge into action doesn't include these sorts of concoction responses. Along these lines, we can make faster modifications between initiation and quieting, like what we can do when we utilize the reins to control the pony.

On the off chance that you go to a canine park, you will see certain apprehensive pooches. They display battle or flight practices. Different mutts will flag a desire to play. This flagging frequently takes the structure that people capture for the descending confronting hound present in yoga. At the point when a canine gives this sign, it prompts a degree of excitement that can be exceptional. Nonetheless, this lively vitality has an altogether different soul than the force of battle or flight practices. This fun-loving soul describes the social commitment framework. At the point when we experience our condition as protected, we work from our social commitment framework.

Injury's impact on sensory system reaction

In the event that we have uncertain injury from before, we may live in a variant of unending battle or flight. We might have the option to channel this battle or flight tension into exercises. For example, cleaning the house, raking the forgets about or working at the recording center, yet these exercises will have an unexpected vibe in comparison they would on the off chance that they were finished with social commitment science (think "Whistle While You Work").

For some injury survivors, no movement effectively channels their battle or flight sensations. Therefore, they feel caught and their bodies shut down. These customers may live in a variant of the never-ending shutdown.

A research focuses on the shutdown reaction through creature perceptions and bodywork with customers. A clarification requires a shiver or shakes to release suspended battle or-flight energy. In a perilous circumstance, on the off chance that we have shut down and an open door for dynamic endurance presents itself, we can wake ourselves up. As instructors, we may perceive this move from shutdown to battle or trip in a customer's move from misery into uneasiness.

However, how might we help our customers move into their social commitment science? On the off chance that customers live in an increasingly dissociative, discouraged, shutdown way, we should assist them with moving incidentally into battle or flight. As customers experience a battle or flight force, we should then assist them with finding a feeling of wellbeing. At the point when they can detect that they are protected, they can move into their social commitment framework.

The body-mindfulness procedures that are a piece of subjective conduct treatment (CBT) and argumentative conduct treatment (DBT) can assist customers with moving out of dissociative, shutdown reactions by urging them to turn out to be increasingly epitomized. At the point when customers are increasingly present in their bodies and better ready to take care of flitting solid pressure, they can wake up from a shutdown reaction. As customers enact out of shutdown and move toward battle or flight sensations, the idea rebuilding strategies that are additionally part of CBT and DBT can instruct customers to assess their wellbeing all the more precisely. Intelligent listening procedures can assist customers with feeling an association with their advisors. This makes it feasible for these customers to have a sense of security enough to move into social commitment science.

Explicit parts of ventral vagal nerve working

The name social commitment framework was picked because the ventral vagal nerve influences the center ear, which sifts through foundation commotions to make it simpler to hear the human voice. It additionally influences facial muscles and therefore the capacity to make open outward appearances. At long last, it influences the larynx and hence vocal tone and vocal designing, helping people make sounds that mitigate each other.

Polyvagal Theory

Autonomic sensory system is about wellbeing. This hypothesis offers exact science to seeing how the vagus nerve, one piece of this framework, which associates the mind, to the heart, to the viscera (the organs of the gut), identifies with our human capacity to interface and speak with one another. Finding out about the vagus nerve enables us to comprehend our sound human sensory system, and how it typically identifies with the upgrades it experiences as fluctuating degrees of security and threat.

This significant nerve is appropriately named by the Latin base of "vagus," which signifies "meander," in view of the broad association it has all through the body. Past speculations clarified that the parasympathetic sensory system, through the quieting impact of the vagus nerve, worked contrary to the thoughtful sensory system. The thoughtful sensory system empowers us for physical activity in the midst of hardship by expanding our pulse and circulatory strain, while all the while putting different capacities like the stomach related framework on hold. This framework empowers us to run from a perilous creature or to act rapidly to manage emergencies without halting and consider it.

The Autonomic Nervous System

This hypothesis gives us a progressively mind-boggling logical comprehension of a three-section various leveled model and how the vagus nerve is straightforwardly identified with a lucid arrangement of correspondence and association inside the autonomic framework.

The expression "neuroception" to allude to our inborn oblivious mindfulness through the autonomic sensory system to impacts in the body, in the earth, and in connections between individuals, at the end of the day, we distinguish perils before we have the opportunity to consider it. This enlightens us regarding the unpretentious feeling of security or risk that possibly influences any association on the planet

The hypothesis depicts the autonomic sensory system has having three subdivisions that identify with social conduct and association. The most seasoned of these subdivisions is the "dorsal vagal," a piece of the parasympathetic sensory system that empowers us to close down, or "solidify" when a circumstance of risk feels wild and we are overpowered. The second is our thoughtful sensory system, or "battle/flight," framework. Furthermore, the most advanced and complex of the subdivisions is our mammalian parasympathetic social correspondence and social commitment framework – the ventral vagus. This is a mind-boggling system of quick, myelinated neural filaments beginning in the brainstem that directs our pulse, breathing, hearing, facial muscles, and vocalizing.

The hypothesis is progressive, implying that every one of the three of these subdivisions pursue a characteristic request contingent upon the perception of wellbeing or threat in the circumstance. In the event that nature is distinguished as sheltered, we are allowed to utilize the ventral vagal social commitment framework, which implies that we are moderately free to act naturally, express our very own emotions, utilize outward appearance effectively, and utilize a regulated voice design. Additionally, our pulse is generally quiet, we inhale unreservedly, and we sift through human language from foundation commotion. However, in the event that we are not recognizing the earth as protected, we fall into a battle or flight, endurance mode (this is the previously mentioned "thoughtful sensory system" dominating). Also, if that framework bombs as well, and we keep on feeling dangerous, we normally fall once again into the solidifying or closing down dorsal vagal mode. In these increasingly crude modes, a significant part of the previously mentioned limits is killed, leaving an individual with far less capacity to identify with the world socially.

Injury and the Polyvagal Theory

With regards to post-horrible pressure, these subdivisions are responding not just to the quick wellbeing or threat in their condition, but also to communication inside between the prompt condition and a feeling of activating action dependent on previous existence occasions. In this manner, in the event that somebody encountered an occasion in adolescence in which they didn't have a sense of security, an occasion in their present grown-up life may resound such an encounter within, and this individual may fall back on the cruder neural frameworks of intuitively expecting to fend off, escape, or shutdown so as to endure.

Every one of us encounters some level of injury in our initial lives. Regardless of whether it was an occasion that brought an incredible dread or we felt a profound absence of help in a huge circumstance, or whether it was a progression of occasions that gave us dread perplexity, or a feeling of not being sheltered. Any of these encounters may have stayed in our sensory systems and develop to add dread to circumstances further down the road that helps our internal framework to remember the peril.

CHAPTER 3:

Diseases and Disorders Associated with Vagus Nerve

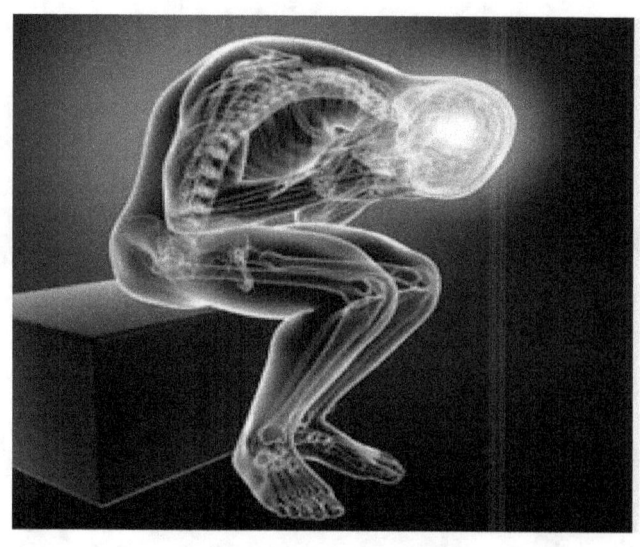

There are different components inside our bodies with numerous capacities. Their performing multiple tasks functions keep us healthy, avoid ailment, and permit the body parts to cooperate consistently as one. One of these multitasks is the vagus nerve. You may have never known about it, however, this nerve plays out a few essential capacities. It is consistently at work. Regularly in the event that you are encountering things like tension, mind haze, weakness, gut issues, depersonalization, and weariness, it could possibly be an aftereffect of a vagus nerve issue.

It doesn't mean this nerve is out to hurt us. Despite what might be expected, it needs our bodies to keep up high usefulness measures. The issue comes whenever aggravated or harmed. In like manner, the vagus nerve turns into a reluctant quiet foe. Before going into the best ten issue of the vagus nerve however, we should discover increasingly about what it is.

Very few individuals truly realize what the vagus nerve is, so first, let me clarify that. Being, the vagus nerve, the longest of cranial nerves in the body that manages the gut and therefore it influence the cardiovascular, resistant, endocrine, and respiratory frameworks. That implies it's an entirely significant nerve in the human body. Therefore, when that nerve is useless, you can envision it can have some entirely strange symptoms.

This past fall, I made sense of that my vagus nerve is, in one way or another broken. What's more, things being what they are, many individuals have a useless vagus nerve. At the point when you battle with vagus nerve brokenness, you can be fit as a fiddle for quite a while, contract a bug, or reach a stopping point, and afterward, your body will take a long time to recoup. I became so ill that I didn't have the vitality to try and get up for a considerable length of time and likely would have shriveled away if my mother didn't bring me nourishment.

Living with vagus nerve brokenness is something that you need to figure out how to live in light of the fact that there is no fix. So on the off chance that you have a companion with a brokenness vagus nerve if it's not too much trouble attempt to get them and read through these basic side effects that accompany it.

Chronic nausea

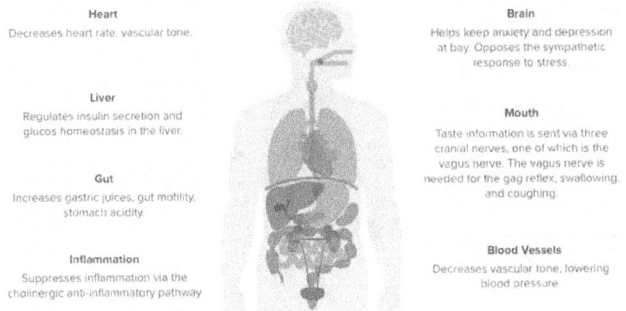

Unfortunately, this implies there isn't a great deal that appears to be mouth-watering to eat. Since you are equipped with more information about the vagus nerve and its capacities, how about we plunge into the main issues it can cause.

With such a great amount going on in the realm of this nerve, tragically, at times things separate.

Vagus nerve brokenness prompts various side effects that many don't have the foggiest idea about the nerve is liable for.

Here are the best-related issues:

- Irritable Bowel Syndrome (IBS)
- Obesity and weight gain
- Chronic exhaustion
- Depression
- Bradycardia and tachycardia (Irregular heartbeat; too slow or quick individually)
- Peptic Ulcer
- Weight misfortune
- Gastroparesis
- Chronic aggravation
- Epilepsy

This one nerve can cause such a significant number of issues. You may be encountering a portion of its belongings and be totally unconscious of the underlying driver.

Knowing a portion of the causes that can prompt vagus nerve issue, can help forestall these issues

What Causes Vagus Nerve Disorders?

Harm to the vagus nerve can be avoided now and again, while in others another infirmity or injury might be the reason.

Providing engine nerve driving forces from the tongue and voice box muscles, just as getting tangible motivations from the chest and mid-region organs, ear, and throat is a difficult task.

Add sending instinctive nerve heartbeats to the stomach and chest organ organs, and throat organs, and there is space for lamentable accidents en route. In that capacity, vagus nerve harm can be brought about by:

Constant Alcohol Abuse

Constant liquor misuse is a whole lot of nothing for the autonomic sensory system, as it has a poisonous, and portion related impact. Strikingly, the vagus nerve is one of those that can be hurtfully influenced by this kind of misuse.

This maltreatment, known as alcoholic neuropathy, makes harm various nerves. Sadly, if a greater number of nerves than the vagus are influenced, side effects can be significantly progressively dangerous for the body's general working.

Diabetes

Predictable increment in glucose can prompt changed nerve science. As this infection can bring about nerve harm to a significant number of them, the vagus nerve doesn't getaway.

Gastroparesis is one of the essential consequences of diabetes-prompted harm to the nerve. In like manner, side effects incorporate clogging, spewing, and stomach swell.

Fundamentally, the stomach and digestive system muscles are never again ready to move appropriately nourishment around appropriately.

Complexities during Surgeries

During medical procedures concentrated on the small digestive system or stomach, the vagus nerve can be harmed. One that is generally connected with this sort of harm is the laparoscopic hemifundoplication. In this manner, this method is utilized as a treatment for gastric reflux.

Diseases

Upper respiratory viral diseases infer another offender as it identifies with vagus nerve harm.

Obviously, it may be difficult to bind if there has been harm at first, as side effects appear to be a standard cold or gentle influenza. Conceivably, they incorporate nasal clog, runny nose, and hack.

Obviously, it becomes clearer that there might be vagus harm when side effects stay for the long stretch.

Subsequently, should vagus nerve harm be the reason, it is spoken to as viral vagal neuropathy or PVVN.

Apparently, a few people experience the ill effects of issues talking appropriately, such as throat clearing, vocal weariness, and diligent hack.

As we plunge further into the universe of the vagus nerve, it tends to be somewhat startling thinking about the manners in which it tends to be influenced.

Consecutively, the uplifting news that we bring means a few different ways to treat the clutters and turn around the harm.

How to Stimulate the Vagus Nerve?

A similar way the vagus nerve invigorates such a large number of components inside our bodies, is the same way it needs some as well. In addition, this keeps the nerve appropriately working and ready to play out its assignments.

In extreme cases, a gadget can be embedded under the skin and takes into consideration incitement utilizing electrical heartbeats. Furthermore, the manner in which it works makes this gadget much like a cardiovascular pacemaker.

Besides, accomplishing vagus nerve incitement comes significantly before an issue emerges. Then again, it occurs if pressure or harm shows up before existing manifestations deteriorate.

Indisputably, a large number of these energizers include things we can undoubtedly utilize in our day-by-day lives. Some may even amaze you.

Methods for vagus nerve incitement:

- Yoga and Meditation - both of these things increment parasympathetic framework movement. Attempt a couple "Oms" the vagus nerve adores it.
- Breathing gradually and profoundly from your stomach

- Exercise-The gut stream is invigorated by mellow exercise.
- Oxytocin
- Positive social associations
- Fasting
- Letting your body conform to cold - cold water in the face, cold showers, and so on
- Acupuncture
- Zinc
- Gargling - gets the muscles at the back of the throat which helps in incitement.
- Massage
- Probiotics - more proof identified with gut microbiota having impacts on the mind.
- Chanting or Singing
- Laughter - can truly be the best prescription.
- Eating Fiber
- Laying on your correct side when dozing

Likely, the rundown comes as a broad one with the end goal that it controls your day-by-day exercises. It additionally incorporates rehearses like straining stomach muscles or hacking, rehearsing Tai Chi which expands pulse and getting some sun.

Eventually, the simple things that we do each day and presumably don't understand, appear to have a huge effect on our vagus nerve.

Medications for Vagus Nerve Disorders

If you accept that your vagus nerve isn't responding to boosts the manner in which it should, at that point your initial step ought to be to get the counsel of your normal specialist. They can prescribe you to a nerve expert that will have the option to decide if you are experiencing a nerve issue.

Experience nerve treatment

If it is resolved that your vagus nerve isn't working appropriately, at that point you should experience nerve treatment. Treatment normally incorporates vagus nerve incitement. A gadget will be connected to the nerve to send electric heartbeats to the nerve to help manage the sign sent by the nerve, this gadget are in capacities comparable to a pacemaker in the heart.

Therapeutic treatment

Notwithstanding, treating the nerve, the individuals who are experiencing this issue should look out for restorative treatment to help manage the reactions that this condition has caused on the body. A conventional pacemaker might be expected to help guarantee that the heart pulsates routinely and prescription is expected to help ensure that your stomach related framework is controlled appropriately.

Chronic illnesses and inflammation

Incendiary reactions assume a focal job in the advancement and industriousness of numerous infections and can prompt incapacitating constant torment. Much of the time, aggravation is your body's reaction to push. Hence, diminishing "battle or flight" reactions in the sensory system and bringing down organic markers for stress can likewise decrease irritation.

Regularly, specialists recommend drugs to battle irritation. Nonetheless, there is developing proof that another method to battle aggravation is by drawing in the vagus nerve and improving "vagal tone." This can be accomplished through every day propensities, for example, yoga, and contemplation or in increasingly outrageous instances of irritation, for example, rheumatoid joint pain (RA) - by utilizing an embedded gadget for vagus nerve incitement (VNS).

The vagus nerve is known as the "meandering nerve" since it has numerous branches that veer from two thick stems established in the cerebellum and brainstem that meander to the least viscera of your belly, contacting your heart, and most significant organs en route. Vagus signifies "meandering" in Latin. The words drifter, dubious, and transient are altogether gotten from a similar Latin root.

In early 20s of last century, a German physiologist named Otto Loewi found that invigorating the vagus nerve caused a decrease in pulse by setting off the arrival of a substance he coined Vagusstoff (German for "Vagus Substance"). The "vagus substance" was later recognized as acetylcholine and turned it into the main synapse at any point distinguished by researchers.

Vagusstoff (acetylcholine) resembles a sedative that you can self-direct, just by taking a couple of full breaths with long breathes out. Intentionally taking advantage of the intensity of your vagus nerve can make a condition of quiet inward while subduing your irritation reflex.

The vagus nerve is the prime part of the parasympathetic sensory system which controls the "rest-and-digest" or "tend-and-become a close acquaintance with" reactions. On the other side, to look after homeostasis, the thoughtful sensory system drives the "battle or flight" reaction.

Healthy Vagal Tone Is the Key Factor of a Feedback Circle Strictly Connected to Positive Emotions

Solid vagal tone is shown by a slight increment of the pulse when you breathe in and a decline of pulse when you breathe out. Profound diaphragmatic breathing - with a long, slow breathe out - is critical to animating the vagus nerve and easing back pulse and circulatory strain, particularly in the midst of execution uneasiness.

A higher vagal tone list is connected to physical and mental prosperity. On the other hand, a low vagal tone list is related to irritation, wretchedness, negative mindsets, depression, respiratory failures, and stroke.

Their exploration recommends that positive feelings, vigorous social associations, and physical wellbeing impact each other in a self-supporting upward winding dynamic and criticism circle that researchers are simply starting to comprehend.

Most researchers utilized a Loving-Kindness Meditation (LKM) procedure, in order to assist members with getting better at self-producing positive feelings. Notwithstanding, they additionally found that essentially considering positive social associations and attempting to improve affectionate human bonds likewise caused upgrades in vagal tone.

How Does the Vagus Nerve Convey Gut Instincts to the Brain? Depended on discoveries by analysts in Switzerland who recognized how the vagus nerve passes on "hunches" of nervousness and dread to the cerebrum, Clinical, and exploratory examinations show that pressure and gloom are related with the up-guideline of the safe framework, including expanded creation of genius incendiary cytokines.

When managed to patients or research center creatures, cytokines have been found to instigate run of the mill indications of melancholy. Along these lines, a few instances of low mind-set, low vitality, and absence of inspiration might be because of raised degrees of cytokine proteins.

As of late, a universal group of specialists from Amsterdam and the United States directed a clinical preliminary, which shows that animating the vagus nerve with a little embedded gadget essentially diminished aggravation and improved results for patients with rheumatoid joint inflammation by hindering cytokine creation.

RA is a constant "Incendiary Ailment" that influences roughly 1.3 million individuals in the United States and costs several billions of dollars to treat every year, as per the scientists.

The neuroscientists and immunology specialists associated with this examination utilized the innovative innovation to outline neural hardware that controls irritation. In one circuit - named "the fiery reflex" - activity possibilities transmitted in the vagus nerve repress the creation of genius incendiary cytokines.

This is the main human investigation intended to diminish indications of rheumatoid joint pain by invigorating the vagus nerve with a little embedded gadget, which set off a chain response that decreased cytokine levels and aggravation. Despite the fact that this investigation concentrated on rheumatoid joint pain, the preliminary's outcomes may have suggestions for patients experiencing other incendiary ailments, including Parkinson's, Crohn, and Alzheimer's.

We can therefore state without doubts that the main investigation to assess in the case of invigorating the fiery reflex legitimately with an embedded electronic gadget can treat RA in people. We have recently indicated that focusing on the provocative reflex may decrease aggravation in creature models and in vitro models of RA . . ., which may be pertinent for other resistant intervened provocative infections also.

These discoveries recommend another way to deal with battling maladies that are at present treated with generally costly medications that have a large group of symptoms. VNS gives medicinal services supplies a conceivably progressively successful approach to improve the lives of individuals experiencing interminable incendiary illnesses.

CHAPTER 4:

Vagus Nerve and Social Engagement

Our Autonomic Nervous System (ANS), is the director of the internal symphony in our body, liable for the control of our real capacities not intentionally coordinated, for example, breathing, the heartbeat, pulse, perspiring, and stomach related procedures. The ANS is continually murmuring at a specific beat, and how well it works, decides our physical, mental, and enthusiastic wellbeing.

The Social Engagement System

The Vagus Nerve is related to increments in wellbeing and passionate prosperity as it produces positive conditions of unwinding and social commitment. Our Social Engagement framework is working ideally when we have a sense of security and associate with the world and others. For the duration of the day, we always get signs and triggers through our faculties and sash, which acts as a second sensory system. We have an outer situation, which is the outside world, yet we additionally have an inward domain, which is the physiology of our body, such as jumping into a remote ocean, so much is occurring underneath the surface, and wave after wave.

Our intuitive inside sifting framework will promptly assess whether we are sheltered or need to make a move. This occurs without us in any event, monitoring it, or contemplating it. At the point when we have a sense of security, we can unwind, grow, go ahead, and step out into the world. When there is pressure or apparent risk in our psyches, we depend on our social commitment framework to set up a feeling of wellbeing and association. This can be accomplished through a discussion, a call for help, looking, or hearing a quieting voice. This will send flags down to our hearts and lungs, hindering our pulse and extending our relaxing. It especially works as a foot brake - a Vagal Brake - and has a quieting and alleviating impact on our sensory system.

Picture the inverse: For instance, an individual says something to you that makes you feel upset. What occurs? We will in general change our outward appearance flagging our agitated, the tone of our voice changes frequently to an angrier, stronger, or higher pitch, we look for approval, and we get the telephone and converse with somebody. On the off chance that the social commitment framework neglects to determine the pressure and it stays dynamic in our body, at that point we will naturally turn to the more established organic reaction, one stage down the stepping stool into battle/flight, with the Sympathetic Nervous framework kicking in.

What are the zones innervated by the Ventral Vagus Nerve?

The Ventral Vagus Nerve innervates the territories over the stomach: face, throat, voice box, larynx, center ear, heart, lungs and serves the social commitment framework. This framework is managed by 5 cranial nerves and when these nerves work well, we can appreciate ideal physical and enthusiastic wellbeing including extraordinary companionship, backing, holding, and adoring connections. At the point when we are socially drawn in, we can be inventive, positive, gainful, and upbeat. Socially connected which implies we are free from dangers, peril, superfluous stresses, and now in great physical wellbeing. The Social Engagement System guides us in direction, correspondence, and outward appearance and involves the accompanying cranial nerves, which all begin in the brainstem.

- 5th Cranial Nerve: this is the Trigeminal Nerve: it is the face and jaw biting muscles.

- 7th Cranial Nerve: this is the Facial Nerve: it controls hearing, center ear, and every facial muscle for informative outward appearances and copy. Neural guideline for the center ear muscles
- 9th Cranial Nerve: this is Glossopharyngeal Nerve: it controls the Tongue, Throat, and Swallowing. It is answerable for sounds delivered by the Voicebox, vocal tone, and making sounds.
- 10th Cranial Nerve: this is the Ventral Vagus Nerve branch. It innervates little muscles in the throat and salivation.
- 11th Cranial Nerve: it innervates the Trapezius and Sternocleidomastoid (SCM) muscles in the neck for head and neck development, direction, and having the option to turn your head.

Practices we show when socially engaged:

- We have a sense of security
- We are associated with ourselves and to other people,
- We can be close
- We contact an associate with others, we can bond
- We are quiet, inhale effectively, and we can think unmistakably
- Muscles are loose
- We feel fun-loving, we move, sing and tummy chuckle
- We feel love and can really cherish
- We can really unwind and unwind into association with others
- Feel the world: it is wide, and we are one with the surroundings

Side effects we can have when not socially locked in:

- We feel on edge or are not ready to unwind around ourselves as well as other people
- We feel shut down or discouraged
- We are overpowered
- We feel outraged, nauseate, disgrace
- We habitually need to do things
- We are wired
- We are antisocial people - don't generally draw in and escape the world
- What do you do? If you don't mind fill in your very own interesting thing you do when you are not socially locked in.

Craniosacral Therapy

The craniosacral system comprises of the film encompassing the spinal string, spinal liquid, the spinal string sac, and the mind. Alongside the focal sensory system, this framework is the most significant framework contained inside the human body.

The spinal rope and the cerebrum contained inside this framework, impact, and help control the focal sensory system. The two frameworks together control body development, perception, thinking, feelings, and wellbeing. In the event that there is a glitch in this framework, the wellbeing of the whole body is in peril.

The spinal liquid that is contained inside the film, known as the meninges, beats at a particular cadence for every individual. As a rule, this spinal liquid heartbeat rate is around ten heartbeats for each moment. This craniosacral beat is like circulatory strain, in that it beats as it moves, both all through the spinal string. Any kind of damage can make pressure be put on the liquid and can interfere with the equalization of the spinal liquid stream.

Whenever the liquid is blocked or can't beat accurately, medical issues are framed. Weight put on the spinal liquid can influence the whole body and cause hurts, torments, issues concentrating, limited development, and different issues, for example, migraines, ceaseless exhaustion disorder, fibromyalgia, scoliosis, and other connective tissue and joint sicknesses.

What is craniosacral therapy?

Most researchers structured craniosacral treatment during the 1970s. He put together his way to deal with recuperation, with respect to standards and hypotheses made by some researchers, who was a rehearsing osteopath during the 1900s. Dr. Upledger went through years rehearsing and consummating his system. Upledger, a biomechanics teacher at Michigan State University, held great and several clinical preliminaries as he dealt with this new method for recuperating.

The rule behind CST is the information on how the spinal framework functions and how the power behind the recuperating functions likewise. Regular stressors can affect the weight of the spinal liquid, just as mishaps and damage. By utilizing a light touch, experts of CST can frequently get the liquids streaming and beating in an ordinary way, in this manner facilitating the torments that a blocked stream can cause.

Likewise, CST can discharge pressures and stressors that are contained in the tissues encompassing the framework. This thusly helps in keeping up with the spinal and cerebrum framework; however, it can likewise work to fix the focal sensory system. By normalizing the beats and the rhythms of the cerebrospinal liquid around the spine and the cerebrum, dysfunctions of the body, for example, incessant agony, strokes, neurological hindrances, and sports wounds can be both reduced and restored.

What are Craniosacral Therapy Benefits?

Craniosacral treatment benefits incorporate diminishing the accompanying issue and issues such as:

- Headaches and Chronic headaches
- Chronic neck torment
- Upper and lower-back agony

- Stress and pressure
- Chronic weariness disorder
- Fibromyalgia
- Post-horrendous pressure disorder
- Orthopedic issues
- Arthritis
- TMJ

Moreover, a great people discover that the treatment is incredibly unwinding. Numerous individuals will in general float off to rest during their treatment. This is in reality exceptionally helpful, in light of the fact that a casual body reacts better to remedial recuperating.

Different advantages incorporate the impact it has on the connective tissues of the body. These connective tissues cannot just apply outrageous weight on the muscles, but they likewise can restrain movement. Since they are not ready to be seen on most analytic pictures, the manifestations an individual displays can frequently appear to be strange and are regularly rejected by conventional therapeutic professionals.

Another part of CST is Somato-Emotional Release, which holds that feelings are additionally part of a bodily injury and that by discharging the horrible feelings, mending is quicker and progressively successful. Regularly, the back rub systems utilized in the CST discharges these feelings. Other treatment benefits incorporate mindfulness of the body and the arrival of the body's oblivious recuperating capacities.

Normally, the customer or patient rests completely dressed on an agreeable couch or unique remedial table. The Craniosacral Therapist at that point tenderly lays their hands on the patient. Most of the craniosacral advisors are osteopaths, chiropractors, rub specialists, or physical advisors.

Subsequent to getting a full restorative history from the customer, the advisor at that point starts with the feet, and utilizing a lightweight, close to the weight applied by a coin being set on the skin, the specialist starts to stir their way up the body of the patient. For the most part, the advisor begins with the feet and works upwards. Notwithstanding, utilizing CST, applied kinesiology is likewise used to help with the reflexive methodology.

CST is a comprehensive treatment, since it attempts to avoid and fix ailment and malady by utilizing the body in general. Specialists who practice CST are commonly delicate professionals who tune in to their patients.

CHAPTER 5:

Tapping into the Power of the Vagus Nerve

Did you realize that constant pressure undermines your conduct when seeing someone? Applied neuroscience explore shows that when your mind and the sensory system are commanded by the pressure reaction, you are inclined to a more noteworthy nervousness, crabbiness, negative state of mind and conduct unbending nature.

This is because when focused on, you lose access to higher subjective capacities like focusing, tuning in, arranging, thinking, and the ability to impart adequately. Did you additionally realize that you have the ability to diminish worry in a moment? It's valid.

You can change your experience by changing your breath. Here's the reason.

The Autonomic Nervous System (ANS)

The autonomic sensory or nervous system (ANS), a key player in the battle, flight, or stop reaction, has for quite some time been proposed to impact social conduct, its capacity is to react to ecological requests by either catalyzing the mind-body framework in light of the danger or keeping up homeostatic equalization during which rest, fix, and development are conceivable. The ANS is isolated into two significant branches: the thoughtful sensory nervous system (SNS) and the parasympathetic sensory system (PNS).

The SNS is frequently likened to a physiological "gas pedal." When a creature sees risk, the SNS dumps a course of stress hormones into the circulation system that expansion pulse, circulatory strain, and breath, contract muscle, and discourage all unimportant capacities like processing.

In this express, the mind's dread hardware, which dwells in the limbic framework, is likewise predominant, drawing significant assets from the prefrontal cortex and different areas of the cerebrum where arranging, thinking and powerful correspondence happen. At the point when the SNS is predominant, social conduct gets constrained to endurance techniques, for example, animosity, shirking, or withdrawal.

The offset to the SNS, the PNS, is regularly thought of as a physiological "brake pedal." Under state of wellbeing, the PNS starts an unwinding reaction, which discourages pulse, circulatory strain, and breath lessens muscle tone/compression and enables the living being to take part in reparative and helpful capacities, an example is in absorption. In this express, the cerebrum's dread hardware is never again activated, opening up higher request subjective working and empowering a more extensive and increasingly adaptable scope of conduct.

The Vagus Nerve

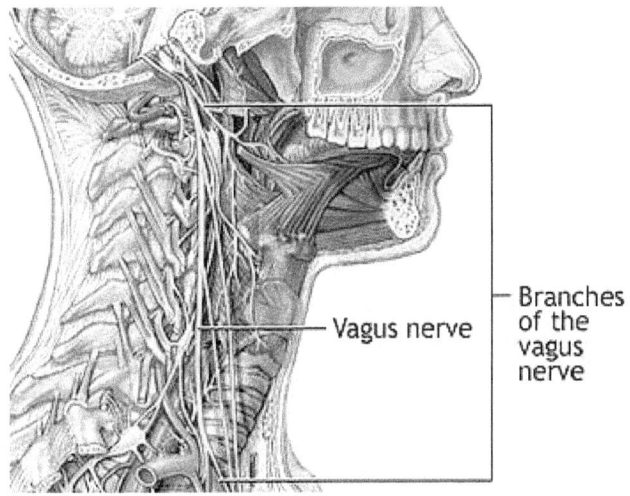

Vagus nerve — Branches of the vagus nerve

Despite the fact that the SNS and PNS contribute fundamentally to our social collection, theory recommends that, for well-evolved creatures and people, the connection between ANS working and conduct is unquestionably progressively unpredictable. Contemporary neuroscientists and clinical analysts are starting to observe the significant impact of the Xth cranial nerve, otherwise called the vagus nerve, in the improvement and upkeep of versatile and maladaptive social conduct.

Charles Darwin previously noticed the vagus nerve and its job in social conduct in 1872. In his book, The Expression of Emotions in Man and Animals, Darwin recommended that the focal sensory system and the vagus nerve take part in a dynamic, proportional trade of neurologic data that influences the unconstrained articulation of feeling. Darwin battled that human emotional articulation is fundamental to endurance, adjustment, and normal determination.

As opposed to being essentially a response to encounter, Darwin conjectured that passionate articulation is proportionally connected to physiology and that particular neural pathways bi-directionally trade data between cerebrum structures and major instinctive organs, for example, the heart, lungs, and gut.

"At the point when the heart is influenced, it responds on the cerebrum," composed Darwin; "and the condition of the mind again responds through the pneumogastric (vagus) nerve on the heart; so that under any fervor there will be a lot of common activity and response between these, the two most significant organs of the body" (Darwin, 1872, P69). This is maybe one of the principal Western logical affirmations of the mind-body association!

The word, vagus, is Latin for drifter. In fact, the impact of the vagus nerve is diffuse. It starts in the medulla oblongata, in the mind stem, and ventures to numerous instinctive organs including the heart, lungs, and stomach related tract, autonomously of the spinal segment. The vagal framework speaks to a complex of nerve branches that hand-off sign from the mind to the body (afferent) and from instinctive organs to the cerebrum (efferent). This bi-directional impact takes into account the productive guideline of metabolic yield because of ecological requests.

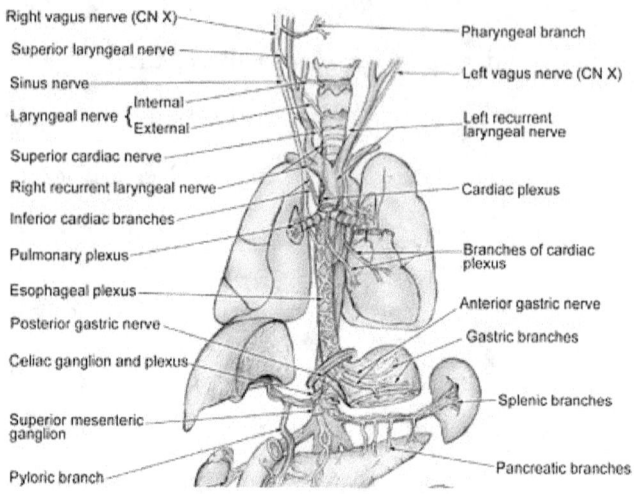

Action of the vagus nerve is alluded to as vagal tone and estimated opposite respiratory sinus arrhythmia (RSA). RSA alludes to the musical increment and decline in a pulse that happens synchronously with relaxing. During inward breath, our pulse increments (thoughtful sensory system impact) and vagal impact diminish.

During exhalation, be that as it may, pulse diminishes as vagus impact builds (parasympathetic sensory system impact). RSA, as a pointer of vagal tone is utilized to look at the utilitarian condition of the parasympathetic sensory system.

In particular, the several number of RSA changeability gives a proportion of the impact of the vagus nerve on the heart. More elevated levels of RSA changeability demonstrate more noteworthy vagal tone during the breath cycle, which additionally mirrors the body's capacity to react to expanding metabolic requests and ecological difficulties.

The view of genuine or envisioned danger enacts the SNS and discourages PNS, or vagal impact. These planned physical responses increment metabolic yield because of ecological requests. When danger is expelled, the vagus becomes predominant and enhances vagal tone increments, starting the instinctive organs' arrival to homeostasis during which recuperation, development, and fixation continues. Stress, at that point, is any genuine or envisioned improvement that upsets homeostasis and prompts the withdrawal of PNS/vagal tone and the inception of a fast SNS reaction.

The main stage, which we find in crude living things, is related to immobilization practices, for example, solidifying and faking demise within the sight of danger. The subsequent stage incorporates SNS impact, which increments metabolic yield and restrains PNS/vagal tone to activate for battle or flight. The third stage, which is one of a kind to warm-blooded creatures, incorporates the expansion of myelinated vagal nerves that are able to do quickly managing heart yield to encourage both commitment and separation from ecological stimuli.

This myelinated part of the vagal framework controls facial muscles relating to talking, gulping, sucking and, in particular, relaxing. It additionally controls SNS pathways to the heart, and can quickly start unwinding quietly. These administrative frameworks of the vagus and related cranial nerves are accepted to give the substrate to passionate encounters and social conduct.

Polyvagal hypothesis interfaces the development of the autonomic sensory system to passionate experience and articulation of vocal correspondence and social conduct. In his times of research, looking at the manners by which the phylogenic advancement of the vagus has influenced human conduct articulation, Porges found out that the more as of late developed, myelinated parts of the vagus nerve found in vertebrates assume a particular job in consideration, self-guideline, correspondence, enthusiastic articulation, versatility to stretch in different limits integral to social working.

These myelinated vagus filaments, which send a sign to the mind significantly more rapidly than the phylogenetically more established, unmyelinated strands, hinder these more established frameworks. Thus the more up to date, myelinated vagal framework in vertebrates can supersede the sign of the SNS, a wonder that Porges alludes to as the vagal brake.

The Vagal Brake and Social Behavior

The vagal brake's fundamental capacity is to direct pulse through the fast hindrance and disinhibition of vagal tone to the heart. At the point when the brake is applied, vagal tone increments and cardiovascular yield is decreased advancing unwinding, self-calming, development, and fix. Then again, when the brake is discharged, the SNS gets predominant, and pulse increments to catalyze the framework in light of ecological requests. At the point when this brake is disabled in any way, shape or form, phylogenetically more seasoned autonomic reactions are initiated, bringing about a limited collection of battle or flight practices.

As indicated by defenders of the polyvagal hypothesis, the vagal brake assumes a significant job in the advancement of fitting social conduct. In view of its ability to quickly discourage or enroll the SNS because of ecological requests, the brake considers prompt commitment and separation from others during social cooperation.

In various investigations with babies and little youngsters, thinks about the show that vagal tone is a significant pointer of self-guideline, continued consideration, versatility and the capacity to quiet down subsequent to encountering a stressor. This ability to control conduct is a fundamentally significant capacity seeing someone. The individuals who can think and act deftly, keep up attentional control, and manage feelings and practices are unquestionably progressively ready to react properly to relational stressors and requests than the individuals who come up short on these capabilities.

Connecting the Vagus, Breath and Social Behavior

The vagus nerve is bi-directionally impacted, both in sending and accepting signs between the mind and instinctive organs. At the point when the body encounters physical or mental pressure, the vagus is selected in the inception of a compensatory conduct reaction by either applying or discharging the vagal brake. Yet, when genuine pressure is ceaseless, homeostatic equalization is troublesome if certainly feasible. The SNS turns out to be reliably predominant and the vagal brake is less every now and again applied.

The vagus nerve controls muscles related to talking, gulping, sucking and, above all, relaxing. It is characteristically connected to social conduct through its enactment of the muscles of the face and neck including those that affect outward appearance and vocal reverberation. Higher conditions of vagal tone and the ability to adequately utilize the vagal brake are connected to more noteworthy enthusiastic dependability, intellectual adaptability, conduct guideline, prosody of discourse, and suitable outward appearance - every single key limit of socially talented conduct. On the other hand, poor vagal brake guideline is connected to broken conduct.

Notwithstanding its effect on facial muscles, the vagus, the two controls, and is impacted by breath. At the point when the vagal brake is actuated and the

PNS framework is enlisted, heart and breath rates lower, and the framework comes back to a homeostatic state, which is normally experienced as unwinding. On the other hand, when the brake is lifted and the SNS overwhelms, breath and pulse become fast, and endurance situated practices identified with the battle or flight reaction become premier.

Since the vagal tone the two impacts and are affected by breath, we can increment vagal tone through control of the breath. As you will review that, there's vagal tone increment during exhalation. By hindering our breath through profound, purposeful breathing and lengthening our exhalation, we can initiate the vagal brake and inspire the unwinding reaction very quickly.

When this reaction starts and PNS is predominant, our minds stop to be administered by the limbic framework and dread hardware that constrains our ability to viably think, plan, reason and react to other people.

This implies that we are never again dependent upon a tight scope of protective or getaway practices. Through purposefully extending the breath and dragging out exhalation, we get to the unwinding reaction, but additionally the ability to be carefully present in relationship.

With time and practice, purposeful breathing can be utilized as an amazing asset to diffuse pressure and oversee troublesome or conflictual relational conditions.

Through changing of the body by means of the breath, we have the ability to change our outlook, yet additionally our relationship to other people.

CHAPTER 6:

Exercise and Stimulation

We learnt so far

Being the biggest nerve in the body, the vagus nerve influences something other than the body's physical capacities. Some exploration shows that a sound vagus nerve is imperative to social holding and sympathy, just as our capacity to settle on complex choices. Spiritualists accept that it is additionally the convergence between our cognizant and oblivious personalities, the physical, and the unobtrusive bodies. Consequently, the vagus nerve might be the most applicable piece of our physical body that identifies with our true serenity and bliss.

Obviously, the vagus nerve assumes a basic job in our bodies; henceforth it is additionally crucial to our prosperity. Individuals with hindered vagal movement can experience the ill effects of discouragement, alarm issue, nervousness, state of mind swings and constant exhaustion. Physically, vagal unevenness can bring about peevish inside disorder, heftiness, heart consume, undesirable pulse, and ceaseless aggravation.

Researchers have been leading examination on the vagus nerve to see how it influences our general prosperity. In their exploration, they found that invigorating the vagus nerve with the electrical sign has the potential for diminishing despondency and uneasiness. Researchers likewise found out that vagus nerve incitement can improve conditions, for example, epilepsy, and heftiness.

Vagus Nerve Stimulation Exercises

Individuals with ideal vagal tone are strong under pressure since they can undoubtedly move from an energized state to a casual state. This switches on the parasympathetic sensory system, which is liable for rest, assimilation, and richness. Subsequently, these people frequently appreciate superb absorption, ideal pulse, and great by and large wellbeing.

Tragically, it isn't in every case simple for somebody to turn on the parasympathetic sensory system and unwind. That is because we invest such a large amount of our energy in a condition of battle or flight. This state is represented by our thoughtful sensory system, which floods the body with pressure hormones.

Fortunately, there are many regular and non-nosy ways that you can invigorate the vagus nerve. Here are five vagus nerve incitement activities to assist you with improving your vagal tone.

Careful Breathing

Long, profound breathing is the ideal approach to enact the vagus nerve. Despite the fact that the vagus nerve is as of now engaged with our automatic breathing, when we do it intentionally it improves vagal tone. This, thusly, allows the body to restore.

Here is a straightforward careful breathing activity. In the first place, try to sit serenely in a seat or on a collapsed cover. At that point, pursue this breath design:

- Sit upstanding and close the eyes
- As you breathe in, lift your collarbone and sit straighter
- As you breathe out, mollify and unwind
- As you breathe in, extend the sides of your rib confine
- As you breathe out, mellow and unwind
- As you breathe in, grow the front and back of your rib confine
- As you breathe out, mollify and unwind
- Repeat for 5-10 minutes.

Notwithstanding careful breathing, therapeutic yoga is a perfect method to invigorate the vagus nerve, as it fuses both the breath and loosening up stances. Here are three valuable helpful stances.

Upheld Forward Fold

Sit with legs expanded straight, and overlay forward over legs. Keep neck and shoulders loose. Make a point to help the middle/arms/head with a seat, reinforces or pads. On the off chance that the low back isn't happy, sit on a pad or collapsed cover. Hold for 10-15 minutes, breathing carefully.

Upheld Bridge

Lay level on the ground with legs twisted. Spot feet level on the ground, hips' width separated. Lift hips, and spot a square (or enormous book) under the low back/pelvis. Rest down onto the square. Hold for 10-15 minutes, breathing carefully.

Leaned back Spinal Twist with Bent Knees

Lay level on the ground with legs bowed. Spot feet level on the ground, and hold a square between the knees. Spread arms out in a T position. Take twisted knees over to the other side. Spot another square, reinforce, or collapsed cover underneath the knees in the event that they don't rest easily to the ground. Dismiss head from the knees. Hold 5-10 minutes, breathing carefully. At that point, rehash on the opposite side.

Exercising Meditation

Exercising Meditation is an awesome practice since you can do it anywhere and whenever. It includes very pondering considering doing a progression of activities that you ordinarily do naturally. To begin with, locate a decent area where you can stroll back and forth for 10-15 paces, or where you can walk consistently for 10-15 minutes. Stroll at whatever paces you'd like, separating each progression as pursues:

- Lift one foot thoroughly off the ground.
- Observe the foot as it swings forward and brings down.
- Observe the foot as it reaches the ground, impact point first.

- Feel the weight move onto that foot as the body pushes ahead.
- Continue for 10-15 minutes, breathing carefully.

Meditation - Mindfulness

The Vagus Nerve and meditation are entwined. The Vagus Nerve generally interpreted signifies "meandering nerve." It goes from the mind stem down to the midriff and associates with many significant organs taking an interest in a large number of our real capacities, for example, breathing, assimilation, pulse, and some more. It is personally associated with the parasympathetic part of the autonomic (automatic) sensory system and along these lines assumes a major job in controlling pressure. The autonomic sensory system runs through our bodies naturally without us taking an interest. Capacities, for example, pulse are a component of the autonomic sensory system.

The autonomic sensory system has two branches, the thoughtful, and the parasympathetic. The thoughtful branch is liable for placing us in battle or flight and the parasympathetic branch is answerable for removing us from battle or flight and managing our bodies when not engaged with a battle or flight occasion.

Feelings of anxiety are noteworthy highs, and one reason for that is the marvel of stalling out in battle or flight. For various reasons our sensory systems are stalling out in the thoughtful mode implying that, the progressions that occur in our body/mind during battle or flight are not being settled after the occasion occurs. Subsequently those changes, to fluctuating degrees, remain with us for expanded timeframes. This results in constant pressure, which prompts a large group of physical, mental, and passionate side effects.

Science has given us various apparatuses whereby we can quantify different real capacities to decide feelings of anxiety. One of the best approaches to gauge these feelings of anxiety is by considering the Vagus Nerve incitement. At the point when the Vagus Nerve gets invigorated it affects the parasympathetic part of the autonomic sensory system to leave battle or flight in this manner decreasing pressure. Here's the manner by which that occurs through reflection.

We realize that contemplation, especially care meditation (full regard for the present minute) is powerful in bringing down pressure. Care contemplation is the most examined way to deal with reflection having more than 2500 examinations distributed worldwide with a normal of 200 more for each month being distributed. I believe it to be the center point of the reflection wheel in that it upgrades the various contemplation draws near and can be an independent practice itself. These investigations showed that reflection could build vitality, lessen pressure, slow breathing, decline nervousness, diminish torment, increment bloodstream, and give a feeling of harmony to give some examples.

At the point when the Vagus Nerve gets the sign from these contemplation impacts, it makes an impression on the mind that everything is great, that there is no risk and there is no should be in battle or flight. The cerebrum at that point sends the message to the autonomic sensory system, which invigorates the parasympathetic branch to leave battle or flight and direct the frameworks into balance. This is a case of the Vagus Nerve and the mind cooperating. The mind can send messages to the body and the body to the cerebrum through the Vagus Nerve.

It is intriguing to take note that an element of the body recently thought to run consequently, can in truth be affected deliberately through contemplation. This is significant and it gives us knowledge into the probability of numerous ways that we can deliberately partake in our wellbeing and its prosperity. This is again showing the psyche or body association, and how our contemplations, feelings, and physical sensations are interconnected, and how reflection can aid the smooth running of the framework.

In the event that conceivable, practice your strolling contemplation shoeless. This enables you to see extra sensations as your feet contact the ground.

Yoga and Tai Chi

The vagus nerve can likewise be conditioned and fortified like a muscle, for instance: Massage and back rub oil, knead benefits for vagus nerve, quieting battle or flight reaction, yoga, and the vagus nerve

Back rub: You can invigorate your vagus nerve by rubbing your feet and your neck along the carotid sinus, situated along the carotid courses on either side of your neck. The neck, back and shoulder back rub; or foot back rub can help bring down your pulse and circulatory strain.

Yoga and Tai Chi: Both yoga and kendo increment vagus nerve action and your parasympathetic framework when all is said and done. Studies have indicated that yoga builds GABA, a quieting synapse in your mind. Specialists trust it does this by animating vagal afferents (strands), which increment movement in the parasympathetic sensory system. This is particularly useful for the individuals who battle with tension or discouragement.

Breathing Slowly:

Your heart and neck contain neural receptors called baroreceptors, which identify the circulatory strain and transmit the neuronal sign to your mind. This initiates your vagus nerve, which interfaces with your heart to bring down circulatory strain and pulse. Slow breathing, with a generic equivalent measure of time taking in and out, expands the affectability of baroreceptors and vagal actuation.

The Amygdala

The amygdala is an almond-formed structure situated inside the foremost part of the worldly flaps. It is a segment of the limbic system and known to have an impact in controlling feeling, inspiration, and memory. It resembles a library, putting away the passionate recognitions that happen each time an idea enters our cerebrum. As such, every time we fabricate a memory, we initiate feelings, so we feel our body's response to our musings. The mind's main responsibility is to foresee and control results.

This implies past encounters, direct responses to recent developments, and structure rehash designs. The cerebrum is one-sided toward what it knows, and will pursue the easiest course of action. The amygdala recollects the emotions around every one of these picked ways, which are the Amygdala, vagus nerve, yoga life systems, yoga, and vagus nerve, feelings, and memory, yoga, and amygdala

The amygdala enacts the battle or flight reactions with an expanded pulse and circulatory strain and invigorates the arrival of specific hormones. It gives programmed, fast, and oblivious response to musings or occasions.

The amygdala enacts at whatever point we experience anything through our faculties that helps us to remember the past injury. In this way, the best approach to manage current triggers is to return to the point of the injury, get to the put-away feeling, and discharge it from the body. The amygdala will never again feel an abundance feeling around that occasion, and it will never again be a trigger certain conduct later on.

Hyperactive vigilance is the point at which the amygdala is trapped on top of it of seeing a danger to life and reacting to it. Similarly as with the vagus nerve, we can utilize knead, slow breathing, and yoga practice to reset the framework.

Obviously, this is nevertheless a concise outline of complex frameworks, able to do more than which is portrayed here, and interconnected with different organs, and frameworks in the body. Be that as it may, I trust this has given somewhat more knowledge and comprehension into maybe how and why you respond to specific circumstances.

CHAPTER 7:

Diet and Vagus Nerve

The vagus nerve utilizes synapses called acetylcholine as detachments to hand-off data along its superhighway. Along these lines, for instance, if there is irritation in the covering of the digestive organs, acetylcholine will tell the cerebrum. The mind will ideally enroll and report that this isn't a perfect long haul circumstance for the gut: supplements may not be ingested so well, and the gut covering may turn out to be harmed to such an extent that it can never again effectively keep poisons from entering the circulation system ("flawed gut"). The vagus nerve will at that point send more acetylcholine with relieving, calming directions from the mind back to the gut.1

Nourishments for Making Acetylcholine

Healthfully it might be astute to help crafted by the vagus nerve by giving nourishments that contain choline, so you can make more acetylcholine. Egg yolks are great wellsprings of choline in the event that they are delicate – or far better, crude, as you would discover, for instance, in new, custom-made mayonnaise. If you cook your egg yolks more, they will contain less choline. Offal is likewise a decent source, for example liver and kidneys. In either case, I would prescribe a natural field that encouraged hotspot for neatness and quality. For a vegetarian choice, lecithin granules (for the most part from soya, occasionally from sunflower seeds) are extraordinary to sprinkle onto nourishments and into smoothies.

You can likewise guarantee a sufficient admission of L-acetyl carnitine (in meat), nutrient B5 (in broccoli, chard, squash, sunflower seeds and eggs) and alpha-lipoic corrosive (from red meat, offal or brewers' yeast) to help with acetylcholine generation. Veggie lover and the individuals who eat low measures of meat can absorb L-acetyl carnitine from lysine and methionine: 2 amino acids typically present in the fish and spirulina.

An investigation done at The Feinstein Institute for Medical Research has indicated that the vagus nerve may really be what they call "the missing connection" to treating ceaseless aggravation that can cause an assortment of different issues - like hypertension, headaches, stomach related problems and any fiery related things like joint pain and so on. All without drugs!

Your Vagal Tone

Vagal tone basically alludes to the inhibitory control of your vagus nerve over your pulse. What the investigations presently show is that vagal tone is vital to initiating your parasympathetic sensory system and all that it does. We can quantify your vagal tone by following your pulse in blend with your breathing rate.

Ordinarily, when you inhale, your pulse speeds somewhat and the other way around, and when you inhale out, your vagal tone is then controlled by the contrast between your inward breath pulse and your exhalation pulse. The greater the distinction, the higher your vagal tone, which is in reality great for this situation since it implies that you are more capable than somebody with a bring down vagal volume, to loosen up your body after an unpleasant circumstance.

Why a higher vagal tone is great

Aside from having the option to loosen up quicker after pressure, individuals with a high vagal tone have by and large better working interior frameworks including:

- Better glucose guideline
- Decreased danger of stroke and cardiovascular malady
- Generally lower circulatory strain

- Better absorption because of appropriate creation of stomach related proteins
- Fewer headaches
- Less despondency
- Less uneasiness (they normally manage pressure better)

What researchers have found out is that, the vagus nerve continually screens your gut's microbiome to decide whether there are any pathogenic living beings. And assuming this is the case, it starts a reaction that at that point controls any irritation that outcomes from these remote life forms, which can influence your state of mind, your feelings of anxiety (and your capacity to adapt to the pressure) and your general aggravation levels.

Healthy Daily Routines for Vagus Nerve

Regardless of the healthful ampleness of the suppers and tidbits, it is in like manner imperative to counsel with your essential consideration supplier or a

Registered Dietitian to assist you with distinguishing nourishing needs altered to you.

Day 1

Breakfast:

- 1 serving of cereal (½ cup dry oats) arranged with one cup water or skim milk, 1 cut banana, 1 tablespoon of nut spread, and a scramble of cinnamon

Lunch:

- 1 meal meat move up: Spread mustard on an entire wheat wrap includes four cuts of dish hamburger, four meager cuts of tomatoes, ½ cup of lettuce, and ½ cup of red or green peppers. Firmly fold at that point cut into four equivalent areas.
- 1 medium banana

Supper:

- 1 serving of this Greek stuffed peppers formula
- 1 cup green beans sautéed in a ½ tablespoon of olive oil

Daily Tip:

Make oats medium-term for a speedy, healthy breakfast.

Day 2

Breakfast:

- 1 veggie omelet, likewise not hesitating to change veggies to preferring
- 1 cup of blueberries or grapes

Lunch:

- 1 serving of fish plate of mixed greens: Mix a 5-ounce jar of wild tuna fish with a little avocado, diced carrots and celery, a tablespoon of a lemon squeeze, and salt and pepper to taste. Devour as seems to be, top onto 2 cuts of entire grain bread, or plunge with cut ringer peppers, cucumbers cuts, or carrot sticks

- **1 medium apple**

Supper:

- 1 side serving of mixed greens with 1 to cups of crude spinach leaves, tomatoes, and cucumber cuts bested with Greek yogurt farm dressing
- 1 serving eggplant pizza

Daily Tip:

Get the entire family required for a pizza party! Set out irregular fixings and enable them to dress their very own pizza.

__Day 3__

Breakfast:

- 1 yogurt-filled melon: Start by on a level plane cut the melon into equal parts. Spoon out the mash and seeds, scoop Greek yogurt into the made "bowl" inside the emptied melon, and sprinkle with **nuts or seeds for an additional crunch.**

Lunch:

- 1 turkey sandwich: 2 cuts of entire grain bread, 4 ounces of cut turkey, arranged veggies, as blended greens and cut tomatoes. Smear the bread with 1 tablespoon mustard or olive oil-based mayo.
- ½ cup curds
- ½ cup pineapple pieces

Supper:

- 1 serving mango and avocado plate of mixed greens
- 2 fish tacos with broccoli slaw

Daily Tip:

Instead of obtaining bundled lunchmeat, get it directly from the butcher in the store to bring down sodium content. Bread is likewise a typical wellspring of sodium, so be watchful for low-sodium brands, or if nothing else providing 140 mg sodium or less per serving.

Day 4

Breakfast:

- 1 yogurt parfait: 1 cup plain Greek yogurt, 1 cup crisp blueberries, 1 tablespoon cleaved nuts, 1 tablespoon nectar, run of cinnamon

Lunch:

- 1 serving of cleaved chicken plate of mixed greens: Top three ounces of slashed chicken, two tablespoons of disintegrated low-fat bleu cheddar, ½ cup of hacked cucumbers, 1 tablespoon of hacked walnuts and dried cranberries on 2 cups of a cleaved serving of mixed greens hurled with 2 tablespoons of vinaigrette
- 1 orange

Supper:

- 4-ounces simmered turkey bosom
- ½ cup wild rice and mushroom pilaf
- 1 cup steamed broccoli

Daily Tip:

After supper, walk the family hound, bicycle around the area, or other physical movement to raise the pulse.

Day 5

Breakfast:

- 1 serving chocolate banana protein smoothie: Simply consolidate 1 scoop of chocolate protein powder (or enough for 25 to 30 grams of protein), 1 little banana (solidified), ½ cup milk of decision, 1 teaspoon dim chocolate, and ½ cup into a blender and blend until completely joined

Lunch:

- 1 hot refried dark spicy burro
- 1 cup cubed watermelon

Supper:

- ½ cup flame-broiled asparagus
- ¾ cup flame-broiled potatoes and peppers
- 1 jalapeno turkey burger

Daily Tip:

- Add 1 to 2 tablespoons of chia or flax seeds to the smoothie for included heart-sound fiber and omega-3s.

Day 6

Breakfast:

- 1 serving high-protein flapjacks, beat with nutty spread, berries, and different top choices

Lunch:

- 1 serving smooth carrot and sweet potato soup
- 2 cups blended greens in with 1 cup of favored cleaved veggies (counting broccoli, carrot, and cucumber), 1 tablespoon balsamic vinegar

Supper:

- ½ cup heated coconut plantains
- ½ cup dark beans
- 1 serving pulled pork with salsa verde

Daily Tip:

Appreciate the scraps of the carrot and sweet potato soup by solidifying and warming when prepared to appreciate once more.

Day 7:

Breakfast:

- 1 avocado egg: Slice avocado into equal parts and take out the enormous pit. Split an egg into the made plunge and heat until the egg whites are cooked and the yolk is at an ideal solidness. Sprinkle on with green onions, diced tomatoes, and a bit of plain Greek yogurt. Shower with hot sauce for a little included zest!
- 1 navel orange

Lunch:

- 3-ounces flame-broiled chicken bosom
- 1 cup of quinoa tabbouleh

Supper:

- 1 serving Thai salmon bested onto ½ cup dark colored rice
- 1 cup steamed broccoli

Daily Tip:

Add flavor to the dark-colored rice with minced garlic and other most loved herbs and flavors. Likewise, cook your rice with different veggies for included fiber and micronutrients, alongside making it in enormous clumps for nutritious scraps to begin another week.

CONCLUSION

In conclusion, vagus nerve contributes to such a significant number of functions in our bodies, keeping it as "happy" as conceivably ought to be of prime significance. This doesn't imply that you need to stress over each easily overlooked detail you do. Just as with each side effect that appears as though identified with vagus nerve damage. Rather, watch and partake in those things that relax you and whatever makes you happy. Evade exorbitant drinking and propensities that lead to diabetes or related ailments. As you deal with your vagus nerve, it most likely deals with you consequently.

www.ingramcontent.com/pod-product-compliance
Lightning Source LLC
Chambersburg PA
CBHW072029230526
45466CB00020B/1184